Breast Cancer Quilts

Dr. Judy Elsley

First Edition

Ogden, Utah, USA

Table of Contents

Acknowledgements

It really does take a village to heal a sick person, and I'd like to thank the community of friends, family and health professionals who supported me through this challenging time. Many of those friends are named on the quilts, as are my doctors. They made all the difference.

Sue McCarty, machine quilter extraordinaire and artist, machine quilted all these quilts. I took each one to her, discussed quilting patterns, and she then worked her magic.

Most of all, I'd like to thank Alan Livingston, my husband, who was there every step of the way. This book is dedicated to him with thanks for the constant and supportive love he gives me.

Introduction

"You have breast cancer."

One in eight women in the U.S. will hear those four words at some time in their lives. In January 2012, I was one of them. I'd had a clean mammogram in June 2011, but discovered a lump as I turned over in bed one November night. A sonogram and biopsy later, I was diagnosed with Grade 2 invasive breast cancer. I had a mastectomy of my right breast in February 2012, followed by chemotherapy from March to June 2010. I went through 6 rounds of chemo, comprised of a combination of Taxotere and Cytoxan. I lost my hair and my appetite, I was exhausted all the time, and I was too ill to work. Those are the facts, but they don't begin to describe the emotional journey of my diagnosis and treatment for breast cancer.

Why breast cancer? The answer is unclear, but in my case, I believe it was related to the radiation I received in 1975 to counter Hodgkin's Disease, which resulted in, among other things, a loss of ovarian function. The hormone replacement therapy gave me a "normal" life for many years, but I probably should have stopped taking it in my late 50's.

I coped with my diagnosis, like so many other women, through the support of family and friends, by taking the experience one day at a time. I also made quilts.

Why quilts? Throughout the breast cancer experience, quilting was one of the few activities I enjoyed. There was so little I could do, but I had the energy and interest to cut up fabric, pin it to my design wall, and then sit at my sewing machine to put the pieces together.

Quilt making gave me the opportunity to express how I felt about this intense and difficult experience. I wrote on my quilts as a complement to the visual image I created. I was fortunate in the support of my husband and friends, but there were times when I needed to vent or celebrate on fabric.

One of my doctors pointed out that quilt making was good for me, an absorbing creative activity that distracted me from feeling unwell, as well as from my fears and worries. Making a quilt helped me focus on the present, and gave me something interesting and positive to think about. I do think working with fabric contributed to my health and healing.

I hope that my breast cancer quilt story will inspire you to tell your story in the creative way that feels most comfortable to you as you make sense of the breast cancer experience.

Chapter 1

A Quilter's Story

Fredonia lies just south of the border between Arizona and Utah. "Blink and you'll miss it," is one way to describe it.: Nedra's Mexican, Judd's car repair, the LDS church and you're on the long ascent to the Kaibab forest for your final destination, the North rim of the Grand Canyon. That's where I started quilting in the winter of 1980.

I was newly married to a seasonal Forest Service employee. In the summer, we lived in a 30 foot airstream trailer on the Kaibab Forest. In the winter, we dragged the trailer down to Fredonia where we rented a little patch of ground on the outskirts of town. Summers were full of camping, hiking, river trips, our seasonal work. Winters were long and slow.

So in 1980, I bought a Dover book about making patchwork blocks, borrowed a sewing machine, bought red and blue fabrics in Kanab, our closest town, and started. In high school, I hated sewing. I couldn't figure out how the bobbin worked and curves defeated me. The garishly orange blouse I began with good intentions ended up, in pieces, at the bottom of a drawer, along with a number of other thwarted projects. But patchwork was different. It was small and tidy with squares and triangles, and best of all, the sewing was all straight lines.

My first block of "Rocky Road to California" was a success, so I made another one. And then I was addicted. I spent all my spare time completing block after block, piling them up until I ran out of fabric. Then I sewed them all together, marveling at the overall design that appeared as I connected one block with another.

What next? I had no idea, so I bought another Dover book on making a quilt, borrowed a frame, a friend and a room large enough to set up. We tied that quilt in an afternoon, and I brought it proudly home to the trailer, but there was a small problem. There wasn't room for me and the quilt to pass through the narrow door. I stood outside and fed the quilt to my husband who then doubled it up on the bed. It was enormous, far too large for our tiny living space. It hadn't occurred to me to measure the space or the quilt; I just kept going till I ran out of fabric. I bought more fabric, more patterns, my own Sears sewing machine, and set to work on the next quilt.

Two years later, I went back to school to earn a master's degree at the University of Nevada, Las Vegas, and then a Ph.D. at the University of Arizona. Before I set off for Las Vegas, I made one final bed quilt — a trip around the world design in bright colors to cheer up my studio apartment. Then I put quilting to one side. It had nothing to do with Medieval English literature, linguistics, or the Freshman Composition I was teaching to earn my way though the degrees.

Three years into my Ph.D. program, in 1988, I was giving serious consideration to my dissertation topic. I loved early twentieth century English lit — T.S. Eliot, W.B. Yeats, Virginia Woolf— so I decided to focus on a little known novelist named R.C. Hutchinson. I liked the one novel I'd read while I still lived in England, and there seemed to be no critical work on him. So I read another of his novels. By the third novel, I understood why no one had bothered writing about him. Did I really want to dedicate years of my life to a second rate novelist whose work I didn't much like?

As I left my library carrel in despair, I asked myself what I would *like* to write about. The answer came to me instantly —quilts. By the time I crossed the quad and entered the Humanities Building, I knew I was on to something. I visited my committee, one at a time, to explain my change of plans. They gave me their blessing, and I was on my way.

In her weekly letter to me, my mother asked:
"I can't imagine what you find to say on the subject. When I try to explain what you're working on, I can't even put it in one sentence that sounds reasonable. Please give me a title to hang my thoughts on to."

I wrote back:
"Perhaps you could say that I am writing about the way women used quilts and quilting to tell their stories and express themselves when writing and speaking weren't readily available to them. I am focusing on the process of making quilts rather than the quilts as a finished product in order to draw parallels between the way we express ourselves and the way a quilt is made. The dissertation is really about women finding their own voices rather than speaking the language of a male oriented society. Does that make any sense?"

I'm not sure it ever made sense to her, but it did to me: I was writing about finding my own voice through the metaphor of the quilt. I spent two happy years working on the dissertation, and in 1990, completed it at the same time I took a tenure track job in English at Weber State University in Ogden, Utah, where I have worked for the last 26 years.

I lost the husband along the way, but not my love of making and writing about quilts. I taught a class on quilts in literature, and another on quilting and writing as parallel creative processes. I presented papers at conferences, published articles, and co-edited an academic book about quilts in the context of literary theory.

I also continued to make quilts. Like many quilters, I morphed from using other people's designs to creating my own, and then, about 15 years ago, I started to dye my fabrics. I began with a book, as I had with patchwork. This time it was Anne Johnson's "Dyeing by Accident," an apt title to describe the results of my first efforts. But like quilting, I became passionate about dyeing. I attended a week long workshop taught by Jane Dunnewolde, who introduced me to the idea of "complex cloth," and then a second workshop with Carol Soderlund who taught me how to dye the exact color I wanted.

These days, I focus on melding my love of text with my passion for textiles as I make text(ile) quilts. As you'll see in most of the quilts in this book, writing on the fabric is an integral part of the quilt making process for me. The words aren't merely visual decoration; they tell my story.

Chapter 3
What the Body Knew

I usually start a quilt with an idea or thought I want to express, but a few months before my diagnosis the four quilts in this chapter came of their own accord. I couldn't title them because I didn't know what they were saying.

After my diagnosis, I realized these quilts spoke about cells working well with each other, and what happens when cell division goes awry. My body knew about the cancer before my mind understood.

The first quilt in the series, "Cells Behave in an Orderly Way," (p. 8) is composed of calm greens and oranges. The cells line up, one with the other, and beaded passageways connect one set of cells with another. Everything is working as it should.

"Cells Working Together," (p. 10) and "The Conversation" (p. 12) explore the same idea of cells interacting with each other in a healthy way.

But intensify the orange and green of "Cells Behave in an Orderly Way," and the cells start to proliferate, wanting to break out of their prescribed order: "The Mystery of Cell Division." (p. 14) Things are going awry.

Cells Behave in an Orderly Way

26" wide by 66" long

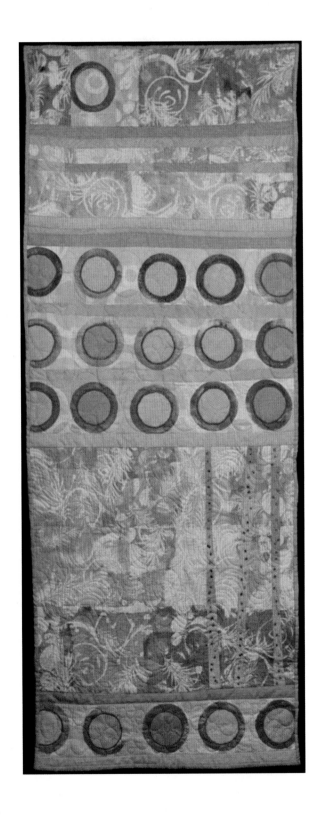

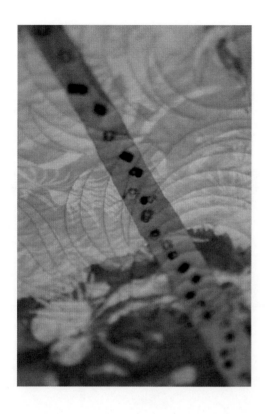

I love adding beads to a quilt. In this case, they emphasize
the connection of one part of the body with another in an
easy and orderly conversation.

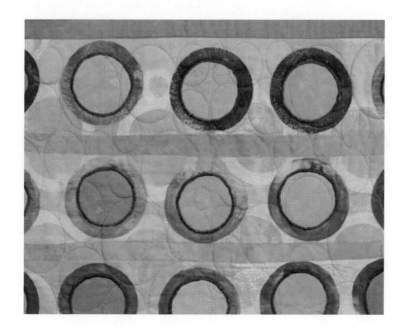

Cells Working Together

14" wide by 24" long

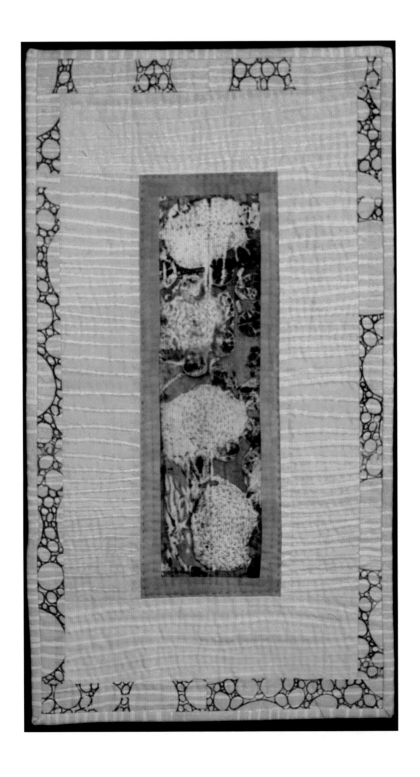

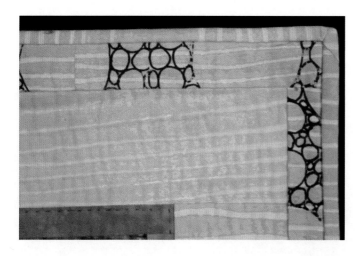

I enjoy the meditative process of hand quilting, the quiet repetition of one stitch after another. However, hand quilting takes an inordinate amount of time. I mostly hand quilted the four quilts in this chapter, but the rest of the quilts were machine quilted by the artist, Sue McCarty.

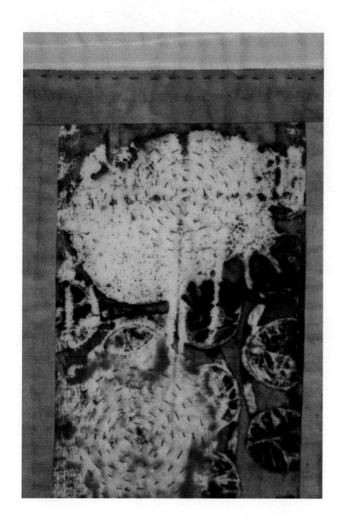

The Conversation

18" wide by 22" long

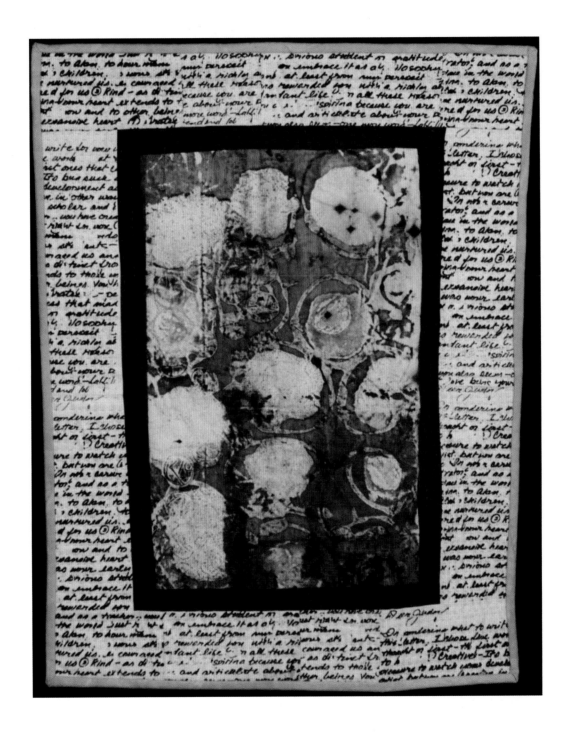

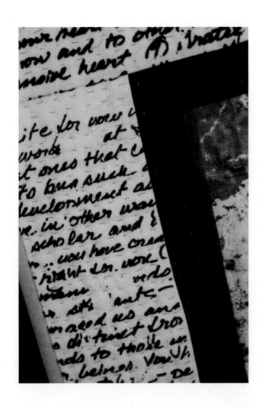

The text surrounding the cells suggest that my whole body is in conversation with itself, one part communicating with all the others to make a healthy life possible. Cancer cells refuse to participate in the fragile work of this physical team work. They act as terrorists disrupting the system.

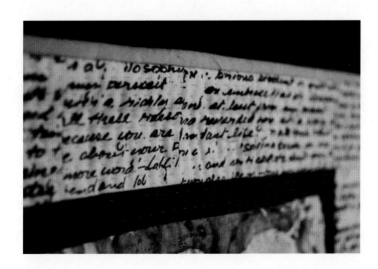

The Mystery of Cell Division.
25" wide by 41" long

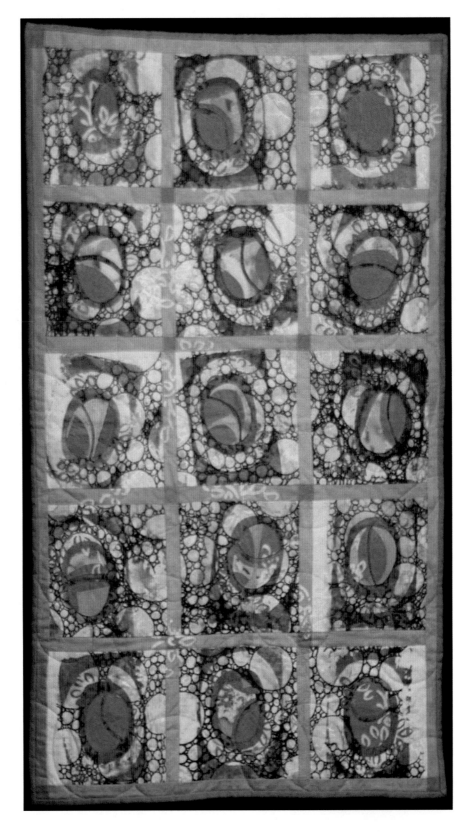

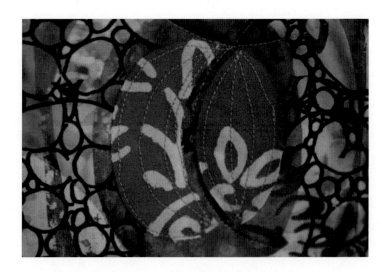

These cells are already dividing, jostling to find a way out of their prescribed borders. They radiate energy and determination. What will stop them?

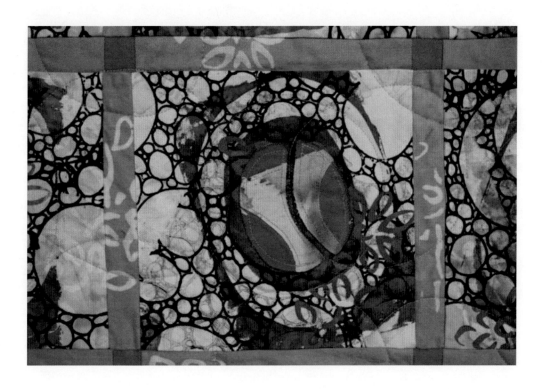

Chapter 3: Journal Quilts

9 quilts: 37" by 58."

In November 2011, a month before my diagnosis, I decided to make one 8" x 8" block of my hand- dyed fabric every day, and then write on it – a fabric journal. This was a way to prepare for my upcoming sabbatical by getting into the daily routine of doing cloth work.

I approached these journal quilts in the same way I write a journal: an opportunity to tell my truth. I wasn't thinking of an audience; I was speaking to myself.

With my breast cancer diagnosis in January 2012, the daily squares became a way to document what was happening to me. As a long-time journal writer, I found I couldn't sit at my computer to write about the experience. I could, however, write a few words about my day on a fabric block. Later, I would sew those squares together.

Eventually, I made nine journal quilts, adding up to 360 days, almost one year. Each completed quilt is 5 blocks across, 8 rows down, 40 total blocks, a reference to the biblical 40 days and 40 nights Christ spent in the wilderness.

At first, I made one block each day, sewing strips of fabric together, with no thought to the completed quilt. It was fun to rummage through my stash of hand dyes, looking for beautiful scraps to include in a block.

After the second quilt, I became more efficient, realizing I was in this for the long haul. I spent two days creating 40 blocks of color coordinated fabrics. This time I cut up larger pieces of hand-dyes, pieces I'd been "saving." For what? Who knew how long I'd live — use that fabric now.

By quilt number 8, I'd run out of my own hand-dyes and was too sick to make more, so my friend, Julie Nelson, gave me some of hers.

The last journal quilt is composed of gel plate printed squares, which I also used for the two healing quilts on pages 69 and 72.

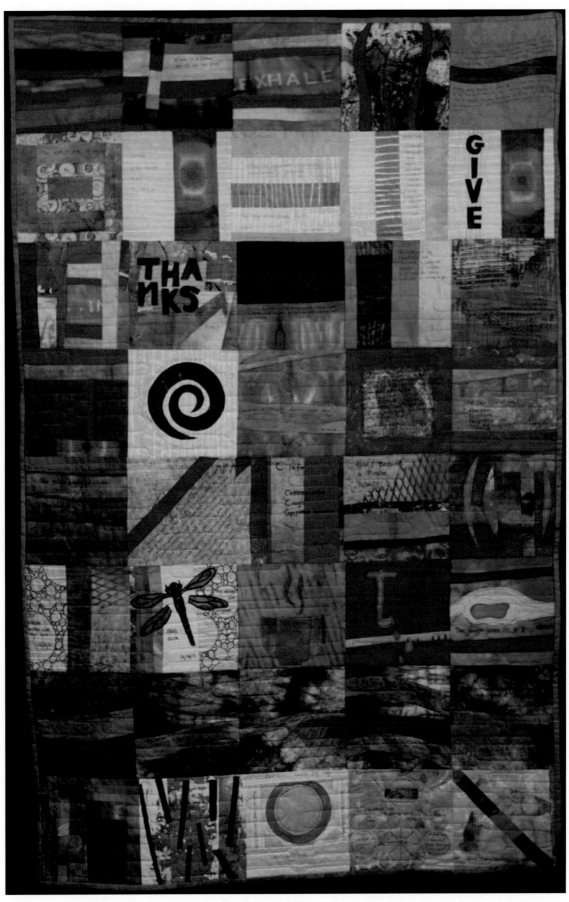

Thanksgiving. I ate too much. I know better. Be present with the first helping so the second helping isn't necessary. 11/24/11

The lights are up, inside and out, the tree is decorated, presents are wrapped. I'm ready for Xmas with only a month to go . . . 11/26/11

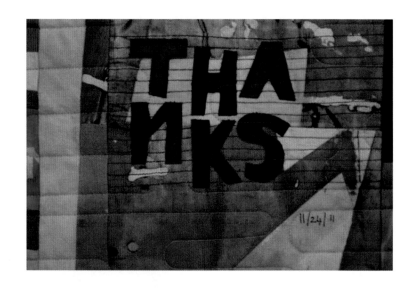

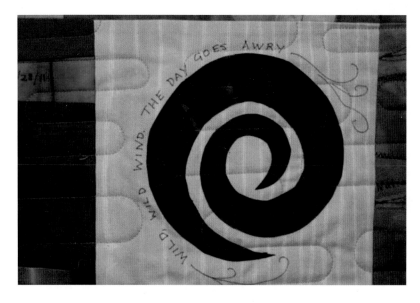

What does illness say? "Slow down, be present, be grateful. Treat this body well." 12/7/11

The rough edges of illness . . . The cough . . . The tiredness . . . Not quite right. 12/8/11

Turning over in bed, I found a lump in my breast. What does it mean? 12/22/11

Wild, wild winds. The day goes awry. 12/1/12

I am recovering from some kind of virus that has laid me out flat for 2 days. "Out of the way," my Body says to the "I" who is usually me. "We have important work to do and you're in the way." So "I" am reduced to a little voice asking for hot water bottles and tea, while my body fights a fierce battle against intruders. The little voice say, "I feel so awful and so exhausted," and my Body replies, "Big deal. Get over it. All you're doing is lying around whining. We're doing all the work. And give us some protein, preferably meat." I have a bossy Body who takes no crap from me. 12/5/11

Journal Quilt 2: 12/25/11—2/18/12

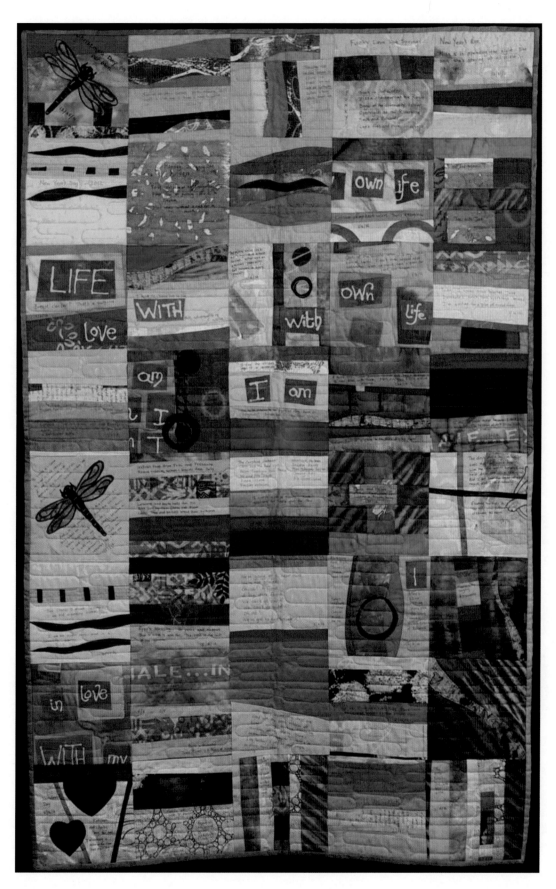

Funky Lava Hot Springs —
Soak in hot water, pizza and
beer at the Royal Hotel, bingo
at the community center. Over-
night at the Riverside Hotel,
and then Lee's fish and rice
when we get back to Ogden.
12/29/11

New Year's Eve:
Kaylee is spending the
night. She says she's
staying up all night. We'll
see.   12/31/12

Breast cancer? That's a surprise. 1/6/12

I have no choice but to live with
this, whatever it is. 1/8/12

Out of the hospital after two and a half
days. Shaky, worried, tearful. I can't think
beyond next Wednesday when we should
have a plan. 1/14/12

Today I would have started Jane
Dunnewolde's week long workshop in San Antonio. Instead I'm
waiting for a plan of treatment.
1/6/12

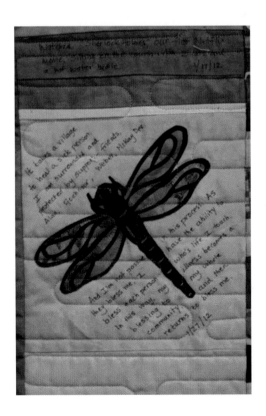

It takes a village to heal a sick person. I am surrounded and protected
by support — friends, Alan,
Gochnour, Weber, MacKay Dee
hospital. And I'm not passive in this
process. As they bless me, I have the
ability to bless each person whose
life I touch. In this way, my illness
becomes a blessing to my whole
community, and then returns to bless
me. 1/27/12

Indian food from Priti and Prasanna
Mashed potatoes, salmon and broccoli from Sally
Lasagna and earth balls from Jill
Egg custard from Gloria
Lentil soup and parsnip bread from Kathleen
Chicken salad and cookies from K
Muffins from Carol, and again from Susan
Carrot soup and bread from Becky

Friends nourish me with their gifts of food.

  1/28/12

"The Constant Gardener"
"Lars and the Real Girl"
"Happy Thank you More Please"
"Mr. and Mrs. Smith"
"Eddie Izzard"
"Downton Abbey"
"Chasing Amy"
"It's Complicated"

I watch a lot of movies. Thank goodness
for Netflix and the IPad.   1/29/12

The days drift by, a buffer until the real work
begins. Like the flat water before Lava Rapids,
these days are calm and quiet. But I can hear
the roar of the rapid and I'm gradually floating
towards it. The only way forward is through the
rapid.   1/31/12

This illness is about community. I am not a passive victim.
I am an active participant in a community process.   2/2/12

Ryan's Mormon blessing: for
peace and support. That is
what I ask for. The rest is the
will of the Universe.   2/3/12

We're going on a bear hunt.
We're not scared.
Oh-oh! A forest!
A big, dark forest.
We can't go over it.
We can't go under it.
Oh no!
We've got to go through it!

2/4/12

Monday, February 6th, 2012

Mastectomy surgery
45 minutes.
Dr. Hansler: surgeon
Dr. Reinhart: anesthesiologist

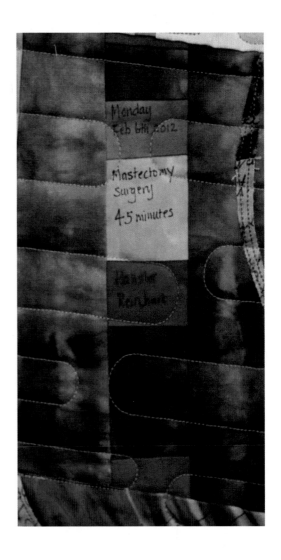

Like baby Holden, my days are filled with
the basic minutiae of living: eating,
sleeping, showering, walking, peeing,
shitting. There's neither time nor energy
for anything else. Like Holden, I rely on
other people to meet my needs. 2/10/12

Follow up with Dr. Hansler. Report on the breast
cancer pathology. Drain removed. The whole day
draining. 2/15/12

This is a gift. I just don't understand how yet. 2/16/12

Whatever happens, it will be OK. 2/17/12

Journal Quilt 3: 2/19/12—3/29/12

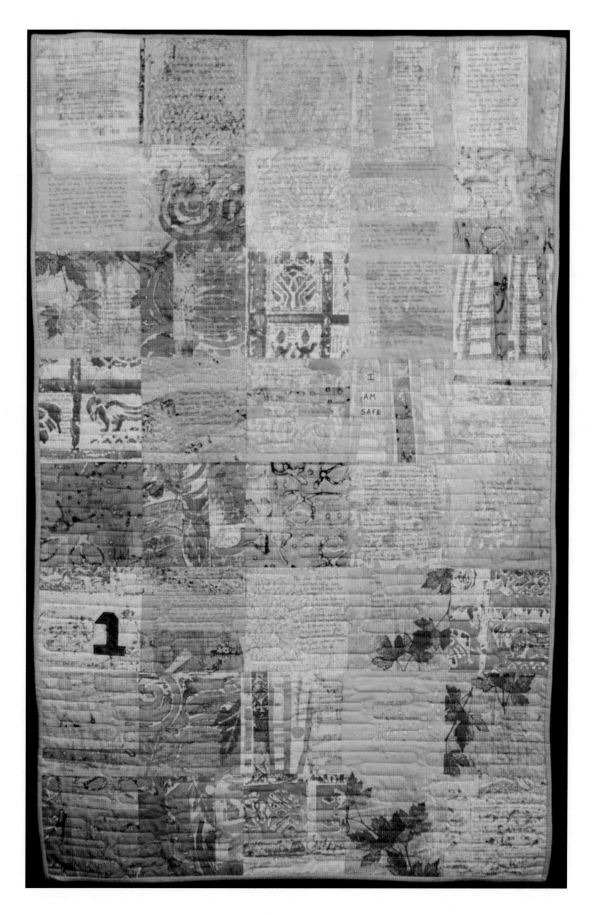

The timing is impeccable: diagnosis at the very start of my sabbatical, giving me months to deal with this. How kind of the Universe to protect me with time, health insurance and a regular pay check. The timing helps me realize that this is as it should be. I don't know why, but the Universe, which gently and lovingly guides my life, sees the bigger picture. 2/20/12

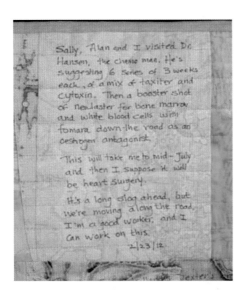

Sally, Alan and I visited Dr. Hansen, the chemo man. He's suggesting 6 series of 3 weeks each, a mix of taxiter and cytoxin. Then a booster shot — nenlaster for bone marrow and white blood cells with formara down the road as an estrogen antagonist. It's a long slog ahead, but we're moving along the road. I'm a good worker, and I can work on this. 2/23/12

Mary called from England and used words like, "shocked," "horrible," nightmare." I was surprised by my own reaction: it's not shocking, nor horrible, and certainly not a nightmare. I feel so loved, so supported, so well cared for and nurtured. My days are full of contentment and gratitude. This path isn't my choice, but it's a remarkably joyful journey. 2/26/12

One of the best parts of the day is the first cup of tea in the morning, made by Alan, and snuggling in bed with two cats. 2/28/12

I had my teeth cleaned as a pre-chemo precaution. 3/7/12

The port was put in today. It took all day with all the waiting.   3/11/12

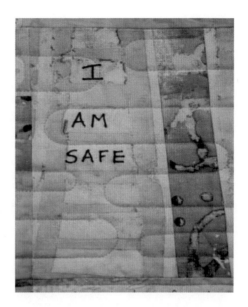

Relationships shift and clarify in illness, like the earth settling after a tremor. The shaky ones fade away, the strong ones come to the fore. Sometimes you don't know strong from weak till the crisis. But mostly, they are what they've always been: what I've established over many ordinary days that hadn't seemed to matter at the time. 3/13/12

Metaphor helps frame the experience: waiting for chemo is like floating on the great lake that backs up behind Lava Rapid on the Grand Canyon. I can hear the roar, but the rapid is still invisible, dropped below our vision. We're almost in the smooth tongue before we see the chaos of white water smashing around our boat. There's no way forward but through, so we cling to the boat ropes as the water crashes over us in all directions. At the bottom, we are sodden, shaking, stunned, exuberant.

Like Lava, I'm waiting to enter the slick tongue of chemo. There's no way out but through. I rely on the skill of my doctors, as I do the boatman, and I cling to the ropes of my life — my values, my friends, my faith in the Universe, Alan — believing they will get me through. 3/15/12

Another metaphor for chemo is the travel we do: China, Japan, Russia, Uzbekistan. First there's the check-in window to make sure all the paper work is in order before we're admitted to security — in this case, a visit with Dr. Hansen. We board the plane in the back room, crowded with chairs and people, little room to move. Our stewards are the nurses who assign us recliners and hook us up to our drugs. We're all on the same cancer journey, on the same plane, but we all have different stories that bring us to this time and place. The plane is confined and safe, like the chemo drip. But what happens when we step off the plane and into a foreign airport? Will someone meet us? Will we safely find our hotel? What will the side effects of chemo be? Will this be an easy trip or a miserable one? In both travel and chemo, it's a series of adaptations to unfamiliar situations; some pleasant, some educational, and some dangerous. It's impossible to assess the trip, the journey through chemo, until it's over. 3/16/12

The Ides of March. First chemo. It took an hour to get to the back
room, and longer to be placed in a reclining chair. The room was
packed. 3 hours but no nausea, just tired. We're on our way. 3/15/12

The other shoe drops. A difficult day of aches, and an unhappy
bowel, no energy. A warm bath was the most soothing solution.

Descent into hell. Body aches, diarrhea. Night sweats, no energy.
Unwell. Ill. 3/18/12

More of the same. Metaphorically, our destination is Nigeria, and I was
mugged the first day we stepped out of the hotel. 3/19/12

I feel like I'm dying. I wish I could die.   3/20/12

I can't do this.
"How do you feel?"
Like shit.   3/21/12

Back to the hospital for hydration. That helps a lot. I cry in the chemo room.
3/22/12

Exhausted and fragile, I re-emerge as a human being. The relief of feeling
normal.   3/23/12

Slow as a snail but in the land of the living.   3/25/12

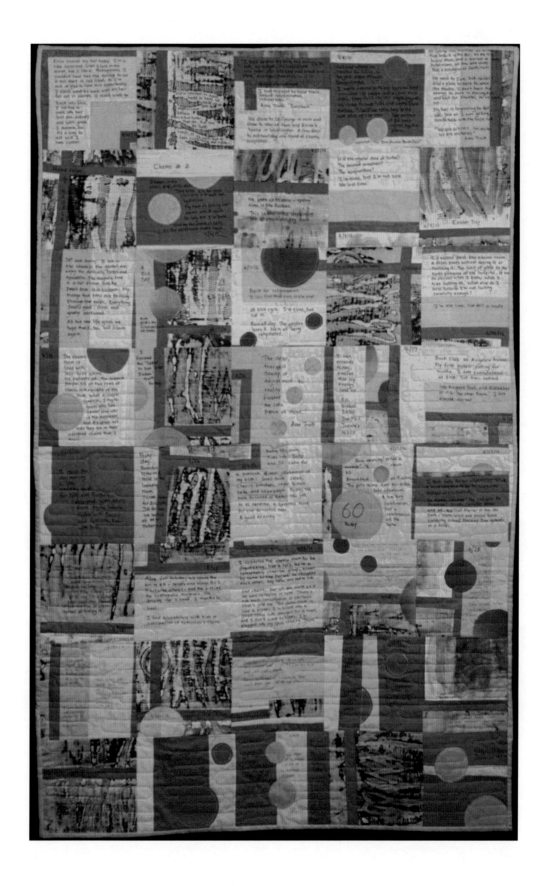

Erica buzzed my hair today. I'm a little surprised when I look in the mirror, but I like it. Androgynous. I wouldn't have had the courage to cut it this short in cold blood, so I'm sort of glad to have this opportunity. I didn't want to wait until my hair fell out in clumps. I didn't want to back into this. I wanted to walk into hair loss proactively and with grace. I suppose, too, it's a way to act as if I have control. 3/30/12

We've learned to walk hand in hand. We could never get the rhythm right because Alan's a foot taller than me. But now we hold hands as we walk and it feels comfortable and right. 4/1/12

We drove to St. George in rain to stay at Shawn and Erica's condo. A few days to acknowledge one round of chemo completed. 4/1/12

My hair Is beginning to fall out, just as I was getting used to the buzz cut. 4/4/12

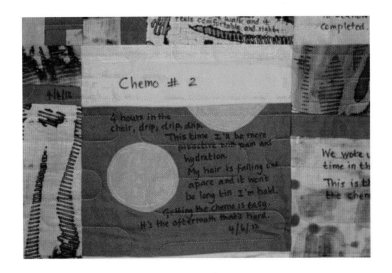

Chemo # 2

4 hours in the chair, drip, drip, drip. This time I'll be more proactive with pain and hydration. My hair is falling out apace and it won't be long before I'm bald. Getting the chemo is easy. It's the aftermath that's hard. 4/6/12

70 degrees and sunny. I sit in the shade in the garden enjoying the daffodils, tulips and hyacinths. The magnolia tree is in full bloom, and my mange touts are pushing through the earth. Everything smells good: fresh and gently perfumed. All this life gives me hope that I, too, will bloom again. 4/10/12

I've walked past the chemo room a dozen times without seeing it or realizing it: the wall of glass on the north entrance of the hospital. It was so obvious when I knew what I was looking at. What else do I miss because I'm not looking carefully enough? 4/13/12

The chemo room is lined with Lazy-boy recliners where we patients sit. The support people sit on two rows in the middle of the room, opposite us. When a couple comes in, I try to guess who has cancer and who is the supporter, but it's often not until they sit in their assigned chairs that I know. 4/14/12

How amazing! What a miracle! To reach 60. Yesterday, a pot luck dinner with women friends. Today, breakfast at Roosters. Alan's girls came for pizza late afternoon. A low key celebration, but a celebration all the same.   4/22/12

I took Sally for a colonoscopy. What a novel pleasure to act as supporter instead of patient. Dr. Porter recited "The Owl and the Pussycat" for us, runcible spoon and all. We lost the car in the car park — chemo brain, and propopel brain wandering around the MacKay Dee grounds in a daze. 4/23/12

Carol Biddle took me to Creative Wigs in Salt Lake City. I hated the wigs: a little white face poking out of a rug. I'd rather wear caps and scarves; to own this time of chemo instead of hiding it. 4/24/12

Pooky day; diarrhea sets in. Even with acupuncture and Lortab, the piper has to be paid each chemo round. 5/1/12

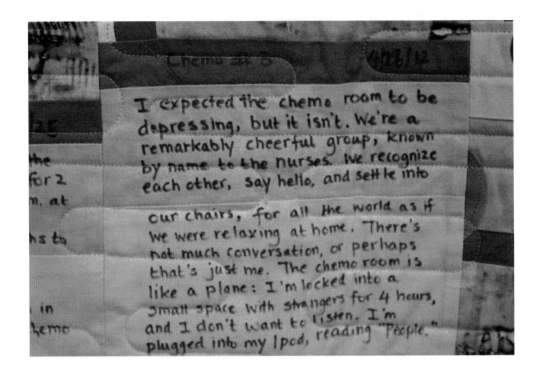

Chemo # 3

I expected the chemo room to be depressing, but it isn't.
We're a remarkably cheerful group, known by name to
the nurses. We recognize each other, say hello, and settle
into our chairs, for all the world as if we were relaxing at
home There's not much conversation, or perhaps that's
just me. The chemo room is like a plane: I'm locked into
a small place with strangers for 4 hours, and I don't want
to listen. I'm plugged into my IPod, reading "People."
4/26/12

Journal Quilt 5: 5/10/12— 6/19/12

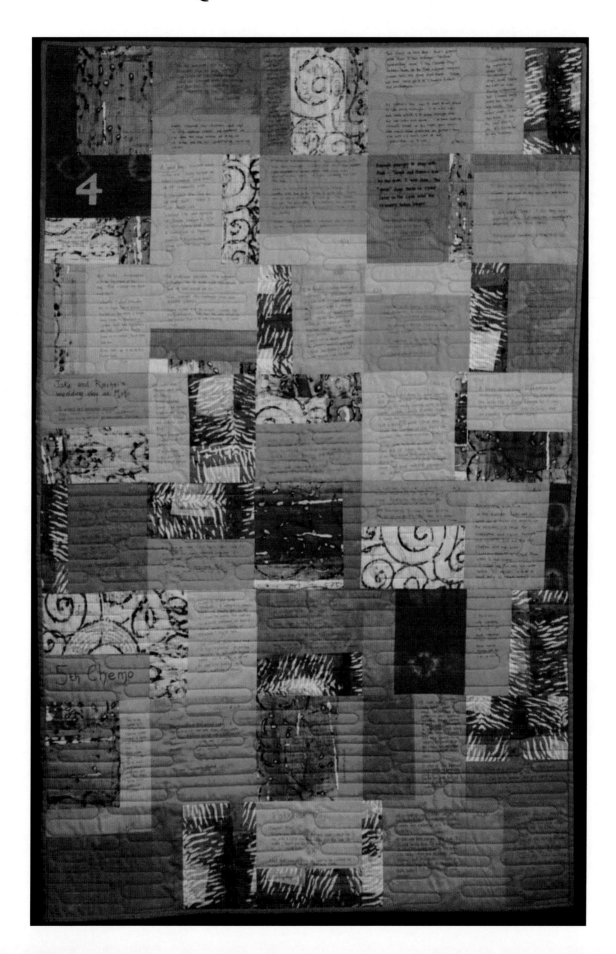

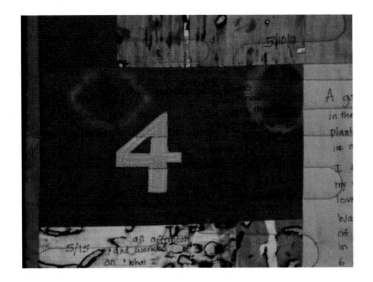

Acupuncture today. I don't mind losing my hair or even feeling exhausted, but I would really grieve the loss of my hands from neuropathy. The fabric work is the one thing I can do and like to do. It's essential to my healing. 5/14/12

Chemo number 4: It seems routine now: the wait, the pinprick to check white blood cells, Andie setting me up, 4 hours of dripping while I listen to my IPod and sew. 5/15/12

The steroids have worn off. I was so pooky today I didn't take a shower, get out of my pjs, or get to my regular meds. 5/19/12

Still pooky. Catherine Z brought me 2 caps she'd made, based on the ones I bought. How clever to construct a pattern and then reproduce the hat.

Finally rising out of pookiness. Coffee with Becky and her friend, Jennifer, and Kathleen. A new person leaves me drained; such limited energy. Jill visited me in the p.m. Such a calm and faithful friend. 5/24/12

Jake and Rachel's wedding at Maho. There are so many reasons I couldn't go: the steps, the sun, the risk of infection, the distance from a doctor. I'd be a liability to the healthy. So Alan goes to walk his oldest daughter down the beach aisle, and I stay at home, fed for 10 days by members of my book club. I heard the wedding via phone, waves crashing in the background. 5/26/12

I haven't read a book in months. The irony of it — an English teacher who doesn't read books. I start a book, but I can't maintain the concentration to finish it. 5/28/12

I'm ready for Alan to come home. It's been a week and the time has drifted by easily enough with fabric work, visits from friends, daily offerings of dinner, naps. I keep the house neat, neat, neat. Not a thing out of place. But now I want the comfort of our daily life together, the companionship. Him. 5/29/12

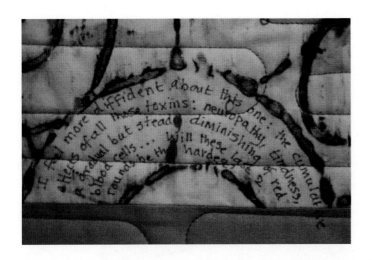

5th Chemo. I feel more diffident about this one: the cumulative effects of all those toxins, Neuropathy, tiredness, a gradual but steady diminishing of red blood cells . . . Will these last two rounds be the hardest? 6/5/12

Zinging along with steroids. A sleepless, manic night. I finally got out of bed at 2:00 am to write the outline for a book on breast cancer quilts. Nutty or possible? We'll see. 6/6/12

Lortab up — 3 X 500 mgs a day. That works to keep the aches at bay. A slow morning. The goal: to eat enough breakfast to take the first Lortab. 6/7/12

Rehydration today. I slept most of the rest of the day. 6/8/12

I have fallen into sleeping day and night. Hard, comatose sleep where Alan has to wake me up to eat and drink. 6/9/12

Acupuncture with Kim. I cried. Why make the effort? Why not just keel over now? No energy. Sleeping most of the day. 6/15/12

Journal Quilt 6: 6/20/12—7/29/12

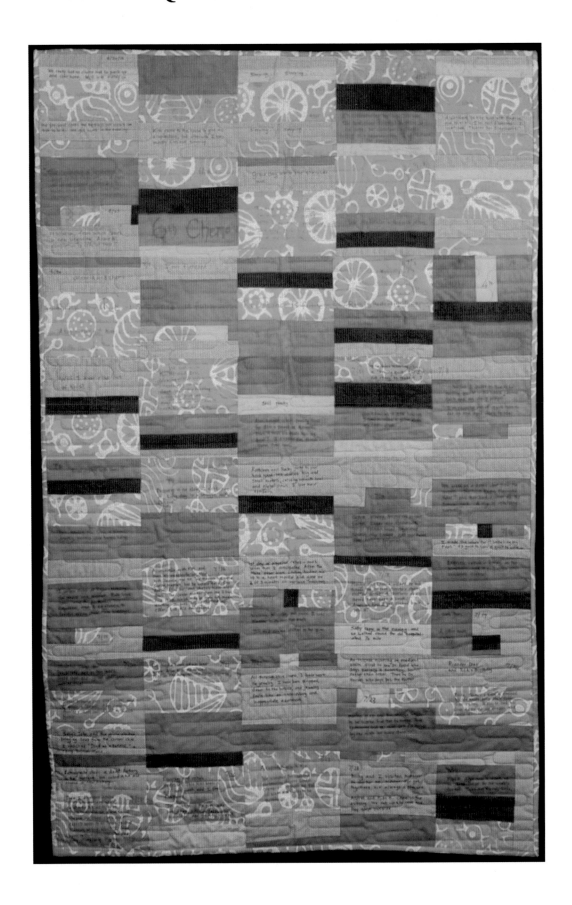

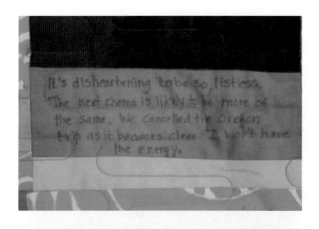

It's disheartening to be so listless. The next chemo is likely to be more of the same. We cancelled the trip to Oregon because it became clear that I won't have the energy. 6/23/12

6th chemo. 6/26/12

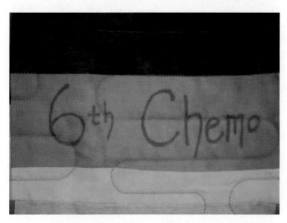

Grace day while the steroids last. The first 3 rounds, I drank smoothies. I moved on to home-made lemonade. This time, green tea with mint seems to work. 6/27/12

Sliding into wet noodle land.   6/29/12

Resistance is futile . . . Resistance in futile . . . Resistance is futile . . . Resistance is futile . . .   Alan feeds me and monitors the Lortab.   6/30/12—7/4/12

Will I ever rise out of this? 7/5/12

We sat with Eric and Becky, drinking water melon smoothies on their front lawn, the evening warm and pleasant. I need more company and I need to start exercising. 7/6/12

Recovery is so slow. I don't see it. Every day is a struggle with fatigue.   7/11/12

1st day of physical rehab — much better than I anticipated. I thought they'd say, "You're too sick; go home." But no. After the intake paper work, Lindsey hooked me up to a heart monitor and gave me 2 or 3 minutes on each machine.

Exercise rehab— 6 minutes on the tread mill, and 3 each on the others. Woohoo! 7/26/12

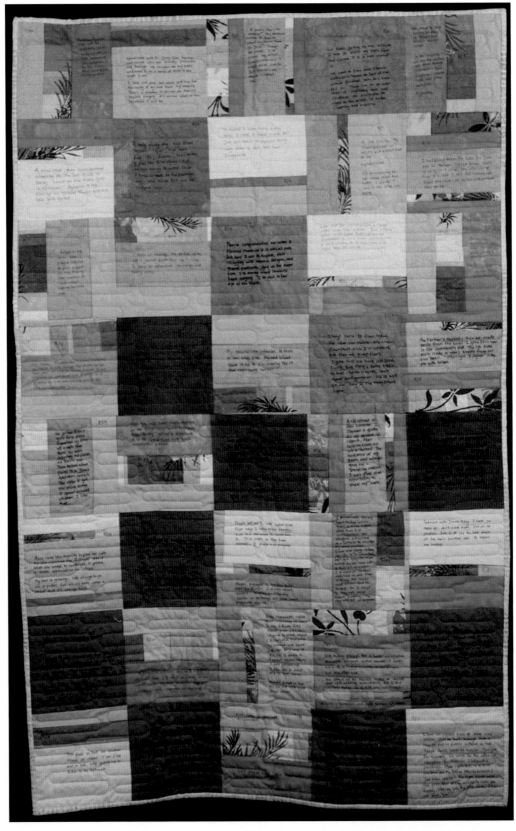

A really pooky day. I feel like I'm dying . Just enough energy to watch
Oscar Pistorius compete on his prosthetic legs, and Usain Bolt win the
100 yard dash. 8/5/12

A low, slow day. It's discouraging to feel worse rather
than better. I wonder if this is the slide into dying.
8/7/12

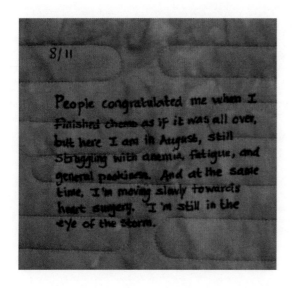

People congratulated me when I finished
chemo, as if it was all over, but here I
am in August still struggling with anemia, fatigue and general pookiness.
8/11/12

My second iron infusion. My red
blood count is up to 11 — nearing
the 12 that represents normal.
8/16/12

Sheryl came to clean today. We have our routine: she cleans downstairs
while I'm upstairs, and then we swap floors. I joke that we have assisted
living: lawn mower, house cleaner, gardener. We're well on our way to the
retirement home. 8/17/12

I slept most of the day. To me, that's discouraging, but Sally says it's
a sign that my body is hard at work rebuilding. 8/25/12

People tell me I look better and Alan says I have more energy, but it's slow. I
can't see it. This feels far from normal. I don't see progress. 8/26/12

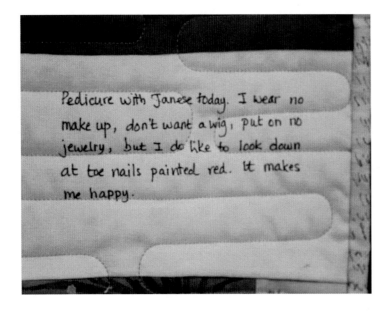

Pedicure with Janese today. I wear no makeup, don't wear a wig, put on no jewelry, but I do like to look down at toe nails painted red. It makes me happy. 8/28/12

Nick's 58th birthday today. Erica and Shawn treated us to a Bonnie Raitt concert at Red Butte Gardens, a celebration of the end of chemo. She was great, going strong at 62, singing one familiar song after another. I've been listening to her music for 38 years. 8/29/12

A third iron infusion, hoping to boost my red blood from 11.3 to 12 or above, in the normal range. It took 6 hours, and I was tired and cramped by the end. 9/4/12

Anita Chernowski called from "Oncology on Canvas" to say I'd won first overall prize ($10.000), first prize in mixed media ($1,000), and first prize by someone with cancer ($1,000) for a total of $12,000 I donate to a cancer related charity. I was gobsmacked. I also get a paid trip to Las Vegas for an awards dinner in October. All for one little quilt about chemo. 8/31/12

I have an overall fuzz of salt and pepper colored hair, enough that I now go out in public without a hat. People don't seem to notice. Tonight, for example, we went to the opening reception for Kathryn Lindquist's paintings. I know I'm in the right place when the president of the university hugs me warmly, calling me by first name, when she sees me. 9/7/12

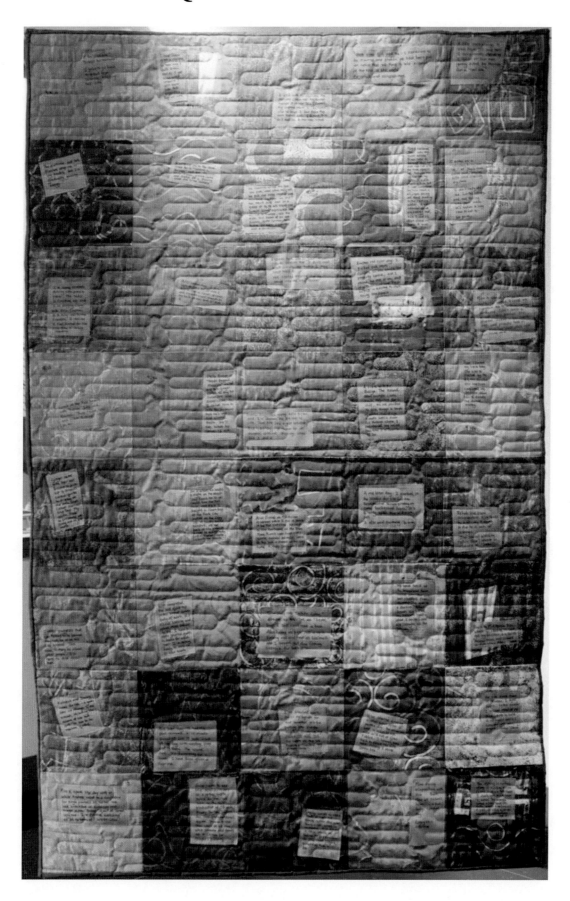

A visit with Dr. Hansen, the monthly check-up. My tumor marker is in the 30s (normal, my anemia count is 13 (normal) and he says I can have the port taken out. I'll see him in 3 months. A reprieve indeed. 9/10/12

The diarrhea and hot flashes stop me in my tracks, but I'm gradually gaining strength. 9/13/12

Casting for Recovery weekend at the Homestead. We learned about the gear, the fish, and what they eat. We put our poles together and practiced casting. We ate too much and met as a group of 14 to talk abut our breast cancer experience. We all live in Europe, so to speak, but some of us are French, some German, some Dutch. So many similarities and differences. 9/15/12

Pam's husband, John, was my guide on the Provo River. A perfect day, warm but not hot, with the first splash of autumn red in the nearby hills. I didn't catch a fish, but I was surprised by how much I enjoyed being out there, wading in the rippling water. I was nervous about my energy level, but I did OK. 9/16/12

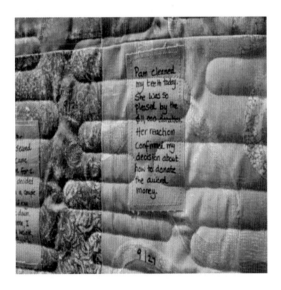

I acted as "secretary to my own life," as Joyce Carol Oates said, paying bills and cleaning off my desk. I am finally off the Lortab entirely and not taking any pain meds. It's taken a long time to get to this point. 9/17/12

I'm running errands, driving from place to place. The radio is cranked up, and I'm singing along with Eric Clapton, B.B. King, Aretha Franklin. I realize I feel normal for the first time in many months. 9/18/12

A red banner day. I swam laps at Ogden Athletic Club for 30 minutes. I had to stop a couple of times, and my arms aren't straight for the backstroke, but I did it. This is the longest time I've gone without swimming regularly in over 30 years.   9/19/12

Ginger came with her son Brooks— she was pregnant with him when she had breast cancer— to pick up 4 cancer quilts to display t the 2012 Utah Cancer Survivorship Day. My quilts, made so privately, are going out in the world. 9/28/12

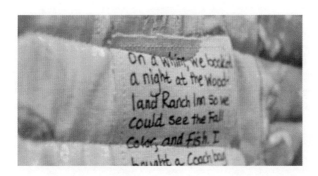

On a whim, we booked a night at the Woodland Farmhouse, where Alan had stayed while I was doing Casting for Recovery, so we could see the fall color and go fishing. 9/29/12

Ginger suggests that the lesson to be learned may not be mine this time around. This time, it may be about other people. I'll have to think about that. 10/3/12

Red letter day: I had the port removed. A 10 minute procedure but it took most of the day with waiting, prep and recovery. The wound is sore. No swimming for a week. 10/9/12

I've started drinking alcohol again after 10 months dry: the occasional beer, a glass of red wine or a tot of Glen Fiddich. I haven't gone back to black tea with milk. Mostly, I drink green tea. 10/11/12

For the first time in months, I dyed fabric. I've used most of my stash — time to build it up again while I consider my next project. 10/12/12

Journal Quilt 9: 10/18/12—11/26/12

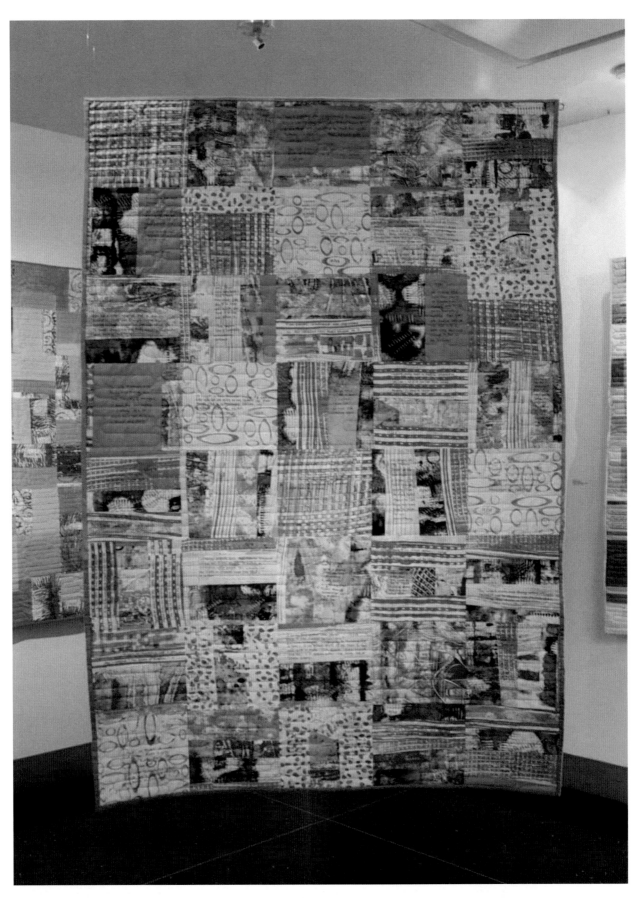

Julie and I met at the studio to dye and play with soy wax batiking. It's such a mess to clean up, and hard to get out of the fabric; I'm not sure it's worth it. 10/21/12

What a surreal experience! Picked up at home and taken to the airport, limoed to the Venetian to celebrate winning the Oncology on Canvas Art Competition and Exhibition. Alan says, "View it all as theater," but all I see is ersatz: fake Venice, fake Grand Canal, fake gondoliers. And it's all about money, extracting as much as possible from the visitors. 10/26/12

Alan has a sinus infection and is now on antibiotics. Julie and I dyed in the studio, trying to make a true black. I stayed for 5 hours, doing this and that, washing out fabric and pulling screens. 10/28/12

Well, that was inevitable — now I have an infection. One day I'm busy and active, the next I'm flat our in bed, ill. This seems like a completely unnecessary setback. 10/29/12

We bought a new Subaru Forrester today. It was time with 168,000 miles on our current car. Even though Chip is a thoroughly likeable, low pressure salesman, we still feel diddled. It's like a casino. You know they're going to win. 11/03/12

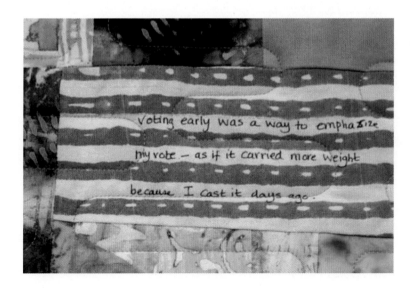

Voting early was a way to emphasize my vote — as if it carried more weight because I cast it days ago. 11/05/12

Election day, and what a surprise and a relief that Obama won. Does the GOP get the message? Rich, white men are no longer the majority. The rest of us spoke up and carried the day. It give me hope. 11/06/12

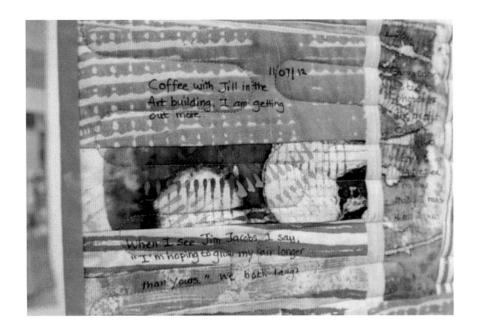

Coffee with Jill in the Art Building. I am getting out more. When I see Jim Jacobs, I say, "I'm hoping to grow my hair longer than yours." We both laugh. 11/07/12

Thanksgiving day at Erica's: we're passing the baton to the next generation. A really good time with Alan's three girls, as well as Alan's ex, Pam, and her husband, Randy. We've come a long way over the years that we can all enjoy a companionable time together. 11/22/12

Tea with Jock. We talked about our aliments and then agreed to change subjects because illness is so boring. 11/23/12

It's just as well I didn't know, when I started the first journal quilt a year ago, what was ahead of me. And here I am, grateful for all the love and support that got me through, and hopeful for the coming year. 11/26/12

Chapter 4:   The Breast Cancer Experience

While the journal quilts gave a "micro" day by day view, the seven Breast Cancer Experience quilts provided the "macro" or larger picture as I articulated visually and verbally how I felt about the experience.

The fabric journal often prompted an idea that I then wanted to express in more detail. For example, I mentioned earlier that it takes a village to heal a sick person, but what did that mean for me? Who was in my village, and what did each one do for me? The quilt on page 50 responded to those questions.

I wasn't well enough to dye new fabrics for these quilts so I picked through my stash of hand-dyes. These quilts gave me the opportunity to use fabrics I'd dyed and printed, but had no idea how to use. "It Takes a Village" was one such quilt.

For other quilts, I turned to my "UFO's, or unfinished projects. Every quilter has some of those, and I had a healthy pile of quilts I'd lost interest in, quilts that were never going to work, and samples I'd made in work shops. This was the time to cut up those orphans and give them a home. "Letter to Sue and Susan" (p. 64) is an example of finding a home for an orphan.

Although I didn't dye any new fabrics, I did print on the fabrics I had, usually with fabric paint, as you can see in "Daily Prayer" (p.56). Other times I discharged color using a bleach gel such as on the "Anna Quindlen Quote" quilt (p.54).

Things I love about this life

52" wide by 64" long

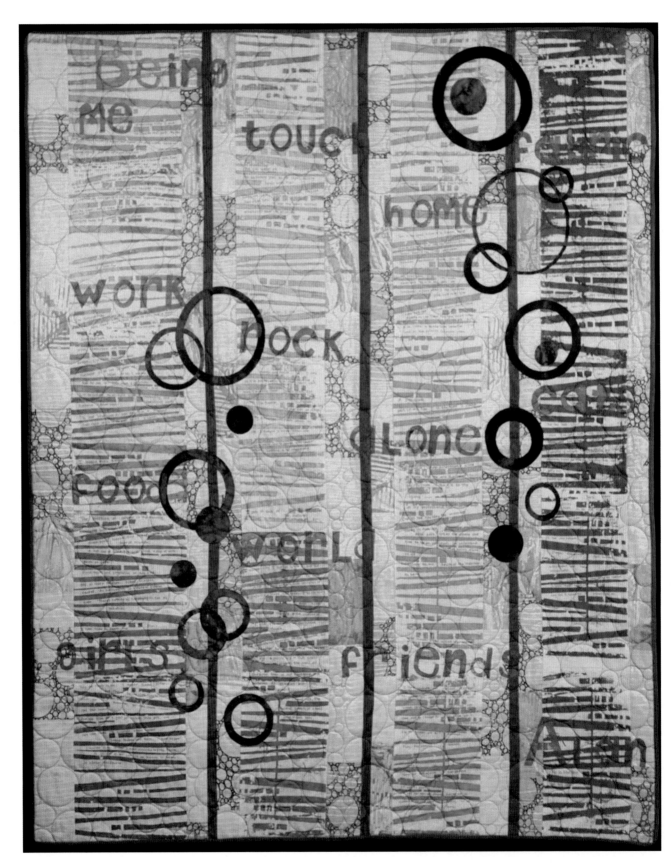

A cancer diagnosis is a shock because it opens up the very real possibility of dying. A good number of times, I've sat in a doctor's office looking as if I'm listening while the voice in my head goes back and forth: Live? Die? Live? Die? That mental conversation prompted this quilt. What would I miss about my life if they were no longer available to me? Here are my answers.

FRIENDS I have sought out, nurtured, depended on, and enjoyed friendships with women my entire adult life. The men come and go (except for Alan, who is my best friend), but the women are a constant: Mary, the various Susans, Shelley, Sally. These are friendships that go back 20 and 30 years. We've had our ups and downs, but we are committed to each other as family. We are family.

WORLD I wonder why I bother with making art when I see the glory and beauty of nature. The best artist can only make a pale imitation of nature's shape and color. I've certainly seen some marvels in the canyons of Southern Utah, the majesty of the Grand Canyon., the understated beauty of the Cotswolds, but it's often the ordinary that catches my eye: a purple iris in full, proud bloom; the grand old chestnut tree in our backyard that performs its miracles each year; a moss covered rock; the twisted branch of a dead bristlecone pine tree.

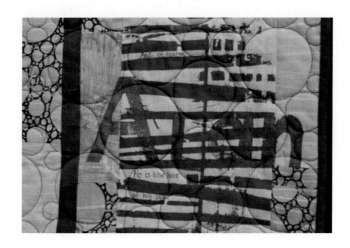

ALAN He is the love of my life.

I have come to deeply love Alan's **GIRLS**. They are family to me. I respect Rachel, Erica and Andrea for the lives they've made for themselves, for their sweet natures and good humor. Pam and Alan did a good job raising those girls, and they have turned into beautiful, strong women. Through Andrea and Erica, I have become Grandma Judy, a role I never expected to play, having no children of my own. I am learning to become an adoring grandmother.

I would miss **PHYSICAL TOUCH.** Foot rubs, hot showers, dropping into the cool water of the swimming pool to swim laps, holding hands with Alan when we walk together. Hugging a friend, the warm sun on my face. I love the many sensual pleasures this life offers me.

I love creating and maintaining a **HOME.** This is the third house I've owned, two of them on my own. I've lived in this house longer than I've lived anywhere, including Shakespeare House. For all its headaches, I do like home ownership. This is my nest, my sanctuary, the place where I can withdraw, filled with things I've chosen with care.

Even at 60, I love **ROCK** music. It's the sound of energy and desire — life! I listen as I'm driving, doing fabric work, when I'm getting chemo. Bonnie Raitt, Eric Clapton, the Beatles, Dire Straits. The list goes on and on. My preferences certainly reveal my age. I thought I might grow into classical music, but it seems tidy and contained compared to the raw energy of rock.

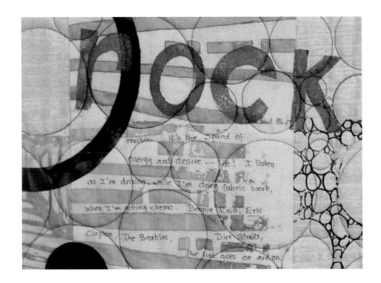

FABRIC work has sustained me through this illness and also through my career: Ph.D. dissertation, publications, classes. And then I discovered dyeing, and a whole new world opened up. I'm passionate about dyeing, and that has renewed my love of quilt making. These days, my quilts are entirely composed of my hand—dyed fabrics.

CATS For the last 25 years, I've lived with cats, starting with Moses, and then Willow. Currently, I live with Betsy and Arjuna, otherwise known as Squishy Bug and Bully Boy. Having cats also means losing them, as we did most recently with Krishna (aka Baby Cakes). I love cats' natures: playful, sensuous, self-serving, independent and affectionate. Cats amuse me and bring me comfort. I know them and yet they are a beautiful mystery to me.

I would miss simple **FOOD.** The pleasure of oatmeal in the morning, sweetened with maple syrup; fresh bread , toasted and topped with a thin layer of Marmite; a hot cup of black tea with just a dab of milk; pesto on pasta; fresh fruits and vegetables of any kind; and, of course, potatoes —baked, mashed, roasted, as hash browns, or in a funeral potato bake. There's nothing as satisfying to eat as potatoes.

ALONE I crave whole afternoons alone at home, just me and the cats. My solitude is the yin to the yang of my very social professional life. One of the reasons the marriage works is that we allow each other the space and time to be on our own. We understand that being alone is as necessary to the health of the marriage as being together.

I love **BEING ME**, essentially since I gave up shame and guilt. My 30's were all about becoming bigger and better; in other words, trying to change myself. But my 40's and 50's were about self-acceptance, loving myself as I am, believing in myself as a beloved gift from the Universe. Who else is just like me? No one. So my job is to become as good as possible at being me, the best me, strengths, flaws and weaknesses included. I even love my beautiful, faithful body. It's seen me through thick and thin, been battered and pummeled over the years, and I hope that I've learned to honor this amazing body that works so well for me.

It Takes A Village to Heal a Sick Person

34" wide by 62" long

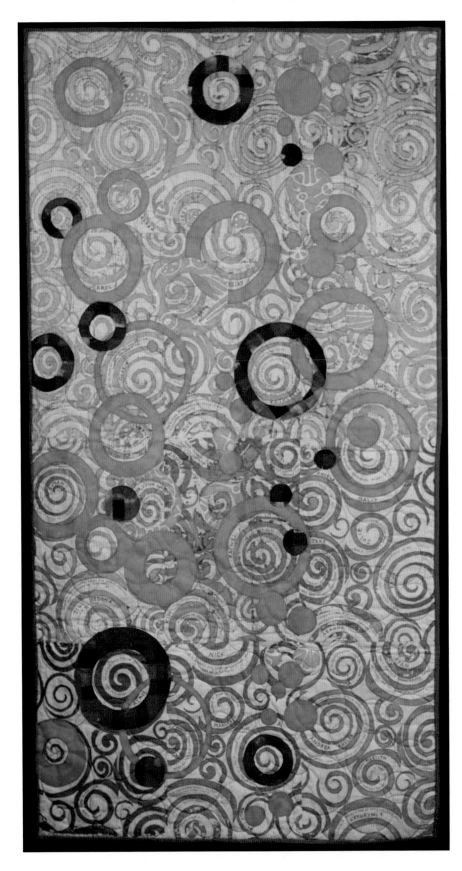

It may be true that it takes a village to raise a child, but it takes just as large a village to heal a sick person, from medical professionals to family members, from friends to rehab support. I've always thought of myself as an independent person, but breast cancer taught me that I am part of a great social web, that my life impacts many lives around me, and that my local community play an essential role in my well-being.

To make this point visually, I selected a screen print I'd made of interlocking circles as the background. I then appliqued hand-dyed fabrics in contrasting colors to make the same point. I used the circles to write the names of my supporters, and what each one had done for me.

The witting is hard to read on the photo of the whole quilt, but this detail shows what I was doing.

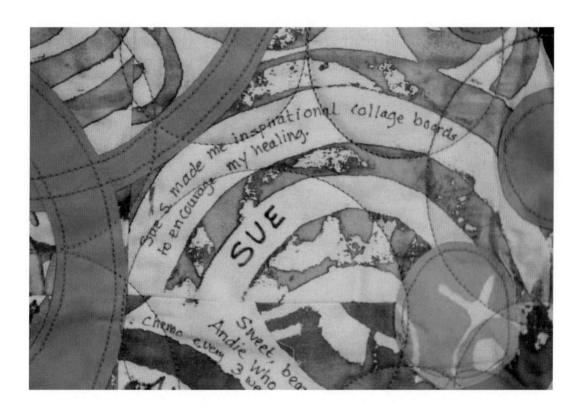

Some people, like my husband, Alan ,were involved all the time in every way. Others cooked me a meal or sent me a card. But for me, every kindness counted, large and small. Every thoughtfulness contributed to my well-being and healing

Here is a list of some of the members of my village, in no particular order:

Susan sent me apricot oatmeal bars she'd baked, all the way from Tucson.

Dr. Gochnour, my family doctor, who takes kind and respectful care of me.

Catherine custom made me hats to cover my bald head.

Diane regularly sent me snail mail cards and put me under the protection of the Blessed Mother Mary.

Linda who brought me chicken noodle soup made from her grandmother's recipe.

Sue who machine quilted most of my quilts.

Becky checked my mastectomy scar and showed Alan how to drain it.

Sheryl cleaned the house once a month.

Kathleen organized sitters for me when I was in the hospital, and then organized members of my book club to bring me food when Alan was away.

Mike made me cabbage and sausage soup at a time when everything else tasted bad to me.

Julie baked me muffins, gave me a hanging basket of flowers, and visited me to share fabric work.

Sylvia brought me classic Mormon funeral potatoes. Yummy.

Eric put me on the Synagogue's Friday night prayer list.

Wangari brought me a meal of delicious baked tilapia and vegetables.

Sally attended all my medical appointments acting as advocate and interpreter.

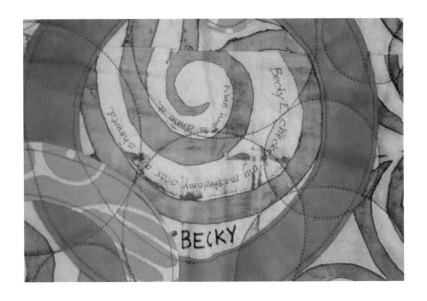

Sue make me inspirational collage boards to encourage my healing . (I used the quotes on those boards in the "Healing Quote" quilt).

Andie, sweet, beautiful Andie, who lovingly administered my chemo every three weeks.

Priti provided lunches from Sitara's Indian restaurant.

Angela, my mother's friend in England, held me in the Light.

Jake made me fabric stamp blocks, mowed our lawn, and fed us when Alan fractured his elbows.

Rachel prompted us all to take part in "Race for the Cure."

Jill made me delicious chicken lasagna and wicked chocolate mousse. She visited me every week.

Sedona made me a pottery mug with my name on it.

Kim administered acupuncture twice every chemo round to alleviate the side effects.

Nick emailed and called me every week, and held me in his heart.

Erica visited regularly with baby Holden to brighten my day.

Andrea and Kaylee visited me, and gave me a JJill gift certificate that bought a lovely summer dress.

Al sent me a box of oranges from Florida.

Kay brought me flowers and chicken salad.

Gloria made me egg custard, time after time; nutritious and easy to eat.

Dr. Joe Hansler did my mastectomy quickly and safely.

Sarah maintained my yard while I was sick.

Corey mowed the lawn once a week.

Dr. Vincent Hansen, my kind oncologist.

Susan drove me to SLC for our Plan B season ticket production.

Alan was there all the time, every step of the way.

Anna Quindlen Quote Quilt

53" wide by 62" long

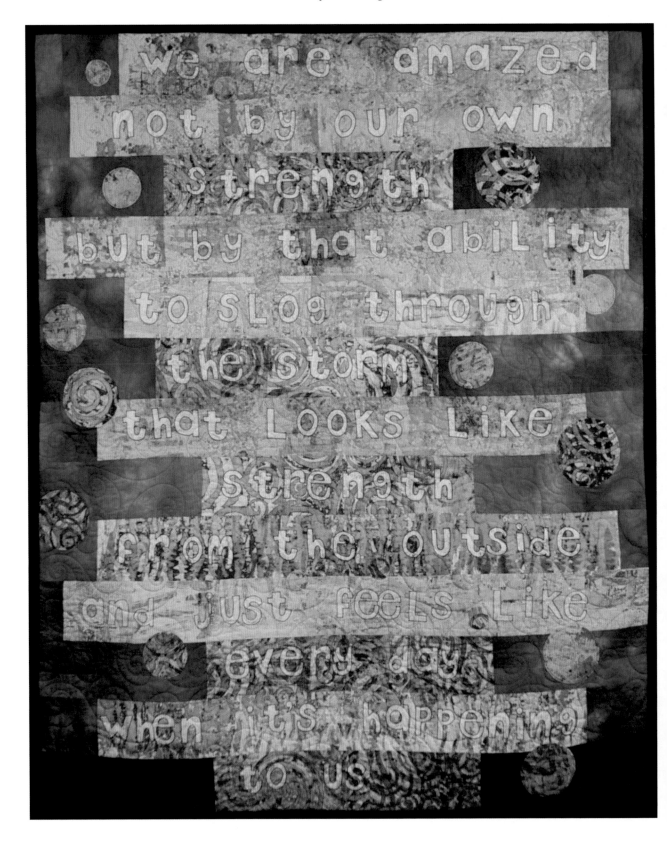

People would say to me, "You're so brave . . . I don't know how you do it." But my experience was not of courage or strength. I struggled most of the time, and felt fragile and weak all the time.

This quote from Anna Quindlen's book about ageing, "Lots of Candles, Plenty of Cake," rang true. She articulated clearly what it feels like to go through a difficult experience, so I transcribed: her words on to a quilt:

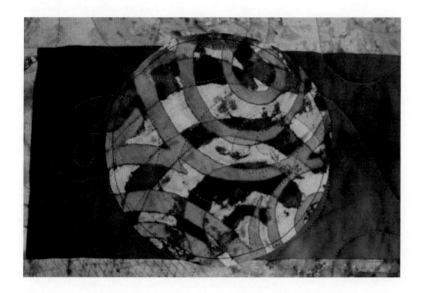

" We are amazed not by our own strength but by that ability to slog through the storm that looks like strength from the outside, and just feels like every day when it's happening to us."

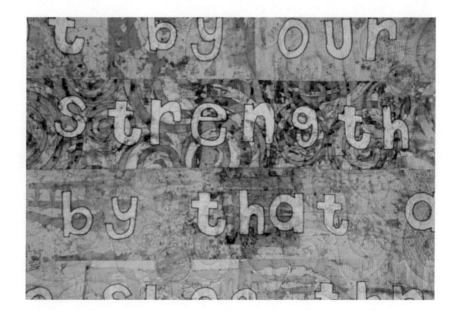

Daily Prayer

41" wide by 37" long

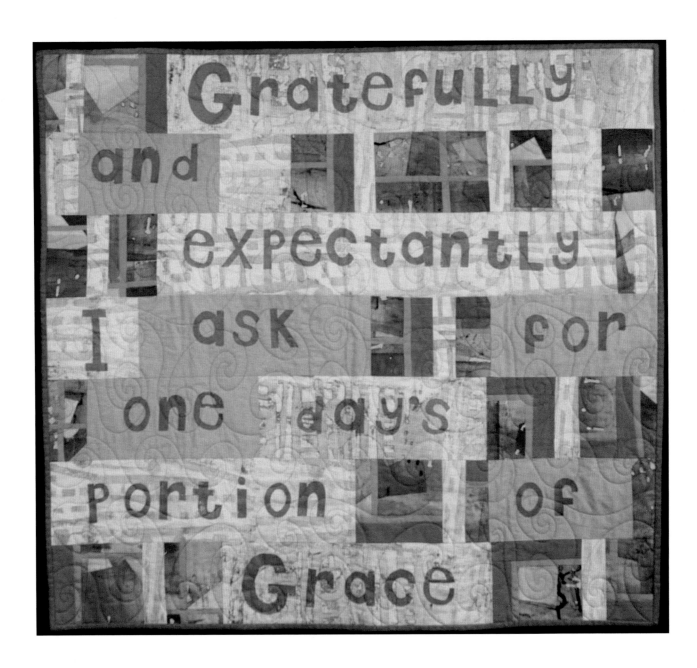

I have come to realize there are many ways to God, each as valid as the next. I was grateful for the Jewish, Catholic and Presbyterian prayers — the source didn't matter. God heard them all. I count good wishes, kind thoughts and acts of kindness as prayers, too. I was particularly touched by the Mormon blessing I received from my boss, Ryan, who anointed me with oil and directed peace and support in my direction. That was exactly what I needed. Whatever happened, I would be Ok if I was at peace and well supported.

I turned my own daily prayer into a quilt, and here it is. Gratitude is so essential to happiness, and at the same time, I am requiring the Universe to treat me well because , as a child of creation, I deserve Grace. What is Grace? So many things: kindness, love, safety, sufficient food and shelter, pleasure , delight and so much more.

Words of Comfort

39" wide by 56" long

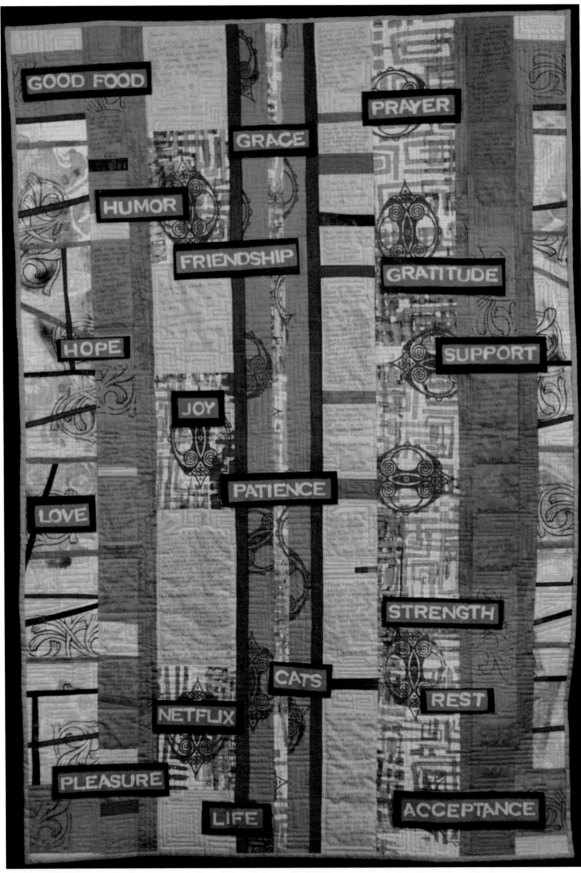

Many people sent me cards or wrote letters and emails to express their support, and I found those words of encouragement helpful. Each one was, for me, a prayer for my well-being and return to health. I have written some of those messages on this quilt as a permanent reminder of the kindness and support of my community.

It's not easy to find good, true words that express support and concern. Most clichés sound lame, especially to the person at the receiving end of them. However, I took great comfort from the thoughtful words of those who spoke from the heart.

Included on the quilt are also some of the ways I coped, from watching Netflix movies to napping with my two cats.

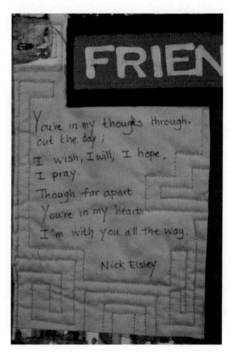

One of my very favorite message of love came from my brother, Nick, who lives in England. He wrote me these lines:

You're in my heart throughout the day;I wish,
I will, I hope, I pray.
Though far apart, you're in my heart;
I'm with you all the way.

My good friend, Dick, who is actively involved in AA, sent me this message:

Of course I am at a loss with respect as to what to say except, "Acceptance is the answer." That is the AA solution to everything over which one has no control (i.e. the answer to every situation). Turn it over. Trust the process, and don't fret about the outcome since you have absolutely no control over it. You can, however, control how you react to it and your note tells me that you are doing exactly the right thing in that regard. Alan's brickness comes as no surprise — he is well trained for this situation. Know that I love you both and my thoughts are with you every step of the way.

Labeling My Fears

28" wide by 37" long

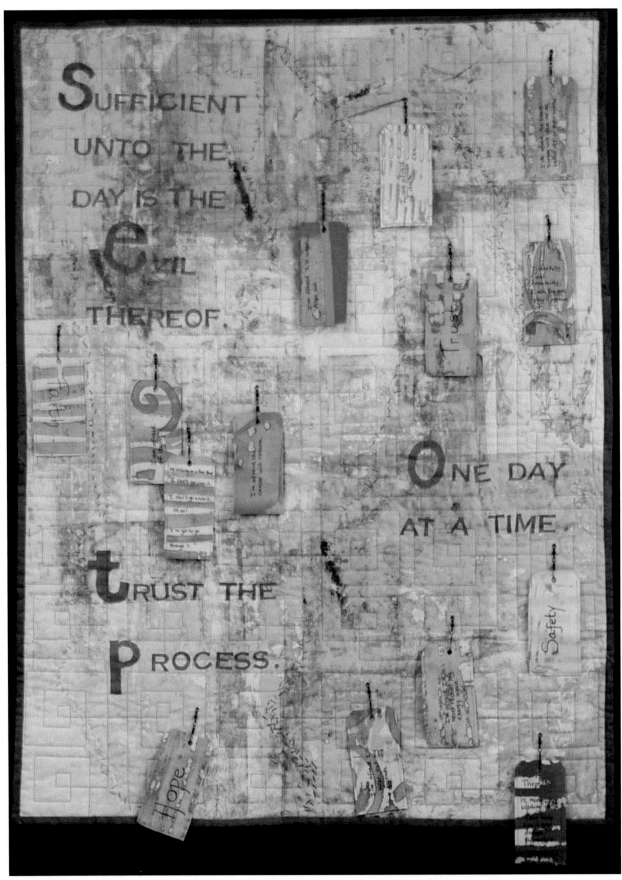

I made this quilt very late in the process because I was afraid to articulate my fears. On the one hand, writing out my fears got them out of my head, but on the other hand saying them out loud made them more real.

The background fabric is a single piece of fabric on which I then printed reassuring words:

"Sufficient unto the day is the evil thereof."

"One day at a time."

"Trust the process."

I have long recognized the frightened voice of the little girl in my head, as well as the wise voice that speaks wisdom. My little girl is named Alice, and she's the one who articulates the fears on one side of each label. Ruth, my wise woman, is a six foot tall Amazon with a thick red braid of hair running down her back. She responds to Alice in a calm and loving way. Alice almost always projects into an uncertain future. Ruth stays grounded in the present and speaks the truth.

I attached the labels to the quilt with barrel swivels, usually used by anglers. The barrel swivels allow the label to be easily turned over to read both back and front so the viewer can read Alice's fear and then Ruth's response. You can read them on the next pages.

A few of the labels bear words of reassurance:

Hope

Courage

Trust

Faith

Safety

Patience

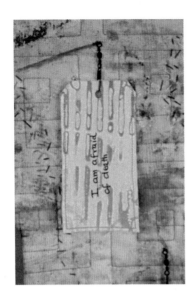

Alice:

I am afraid of death

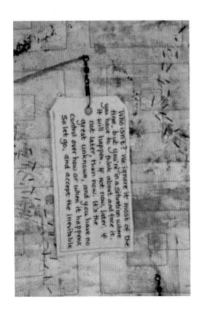

Ruth:

Yes, so is everyone else. Most people can ignore it most of the time, but it happens to all of us. You happen to be in a situation where you have to think about it and face it. It will happen. If not now, later. If not later, now. It's the great unknown, and you have no control over how or when it happens. So let go and accept the inevitable.

I am afraid of dying

That's a reasonable fear. The loss of physical strength, of personality, of life. The process is scary, there are no two ways about it. But Alan is here, the hospital is here. You will be well cared for through the process. It will be a process of releasing this and then that. Letting go as gently as you can.

I am afraid I'll never recover my energy again

After so many weeks of chemo, that's a natural fear, especially these last two rounds of chemo with the accumulation of chemo and then the anemia. But nothing stays the same. You'll regain your energy or you'll sink further, but it won't always be like this. Right now, the best thing to do is rest, eat well, get some exercise, keep sewing, visit with friends. Patience is the key.

I am afraid the cancer will return

It probably will, especially if your current issues are the long term result of radiation for the Hodgkin's. Let's hope that next time will be a good number of years off, and that it will be advanced pancreatic cancer so there's no messing around with chemo and the hope of recovery.

I am afraid that I'll wear Alan out

You chose him, in good part, because you could see he'd be able to help you through illness and dying, and he has done that. It's important to check in with him regularly, to give him plenty of time off, to make only the demands that you really need.

I am afraid I'll wear out my friends

The same is true for them as for Alan. Never play the guilt game. Let them come when they want to. Don't make expectations. Thank them for each kind act. Appreciate everything they do for you. And remember that they want to help.

Letter to Sue and Susan

40" wide by 58" long

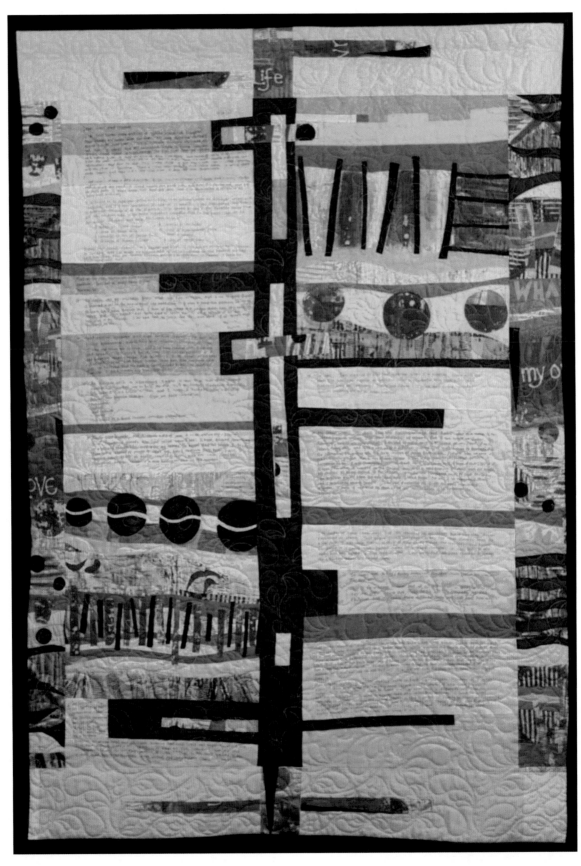

Although I'm an avid reader and writer, and a dedicated English teacher, I could not write about my breast cancer experience as I was going through it. However, I wrote to two friends, Sue and Susan, who I have known for over 20 years, explaining what I was going through. We met in graduate school in the 1980's, and all three of us are writers.

We each contribute to a communal journal that we send to one to the other. We're on our fifth or sixth journal, and the box we send each other always contains very good quality chocolate.

This letter was my contribution to that journal. After I'd sent it off, I decided to inscribe the letter on a quilt as a record of my life at that time. The letter lists all the reasons I'm grateful for my current life.

Friday, April 6th 2012

Dear Sue and Susan,

I'm just home from getting a white blood cell booster that makes my bones ache for days. My bone marrow doesn't want to do overtime: "We're already working as hard as we can." I agree, but my oncologist wants to make sure my white blood count is high enough for the next dose of chemo in 3 weeks time. I had my second dose yesterday; four hours of drip, drip, dripping. First the anti-nausea medication for my brain. Then the anti-nausea medication for my stomach. And then the bad, bad chemo stuff. I get two kinds. One is called Cytoxan, and the other is Taxotere. They're more heart friendly than other drugs. I get a day's grace today, and then if it's like last time, I drop into non-humanness.

Last week, Alan's middle daughter, Erica, the hairdresser who just had a baby, came and buzzed my head. I liked having very short hair, but now it's falling out, and I'll be bald soon. I'm developing a repertoire of hats and scarves.

I'm trying to be more proactive this time. I'm taking the Lortab on schedule, along with ibuprofen, and I'm taking Imodium as soon as I need it. I got dehydrated last time, in good part because of all the diarrhea. I've bought a very nifty smoothie making machine that will help me drink more. I can make individual smoothies right in the plastic cup, so no decanting. It's quick and easy. My current recipe is:

A dollop of Greek yogurt
a slosh of whole milk and a slosh of pomegranate juice
a spoonful or two of frozen fruit
several ice cubes
half a banana
a spoonful of powdered protein
a slug of maple syrup

Doesn't that sound healthy and good? It's yummy. I'll have an acupuncture session on Tuesday, and I've made an appointment to get rehydrated at the hospital on Wednesday. We'll see if my new pro-active regimen makes the slightest difference. I hope so. Last time was hell.

Most of the time, though, my main response to all this is gratitude. There are so many things I feel grateful for:

- The timing. All my sabbatical plans went out the window, but 1 am so glad that I was diagnosed right at the beginning of the sabbatical, and I don't have the pressure of trying to work while going through this. I think of the timing in a larger sense, too. It's amazing, really, that I haven't had some kind of cancer earlier, as a result of all that radiation in my twenties. I've had time to live a full life, do a whole lot of things that mattered to me, and I'm well enough established in my career that there are no pressures from Weber.

- Good medical insurance. The cost of all this is astronomical, and I have dual insurance because of Alan. I don't have to worry about paying for diagnosis and treatment.

- Good medical support. I've liked and trusted my doctors, and I've been treated with kindness and respect.

- An amazing brick of a husband. Early on, I told Alan that if we stayed together, I expected him to help me die. With my history, it's likely I'll die before he does, and I want a partner who will step through the process with me. Alan has been wonderful: Supportive, patient, good humored, loving. This would be a much harder process without him.

- Really good friends, and I count both of you in that category. Loving, kind, thoughtful friends who have rallied around me. I have become something of a recluse through this, harboring my energy for myself and the people I trust. There are a good number of people I won't see, and I pick carefully those I will. I have a small group of trusted friends who are calm, sane, helpful, loving. I'm very self-protective at the moment.

- My fabric work. I don't have the concentration to read books, and this letter is the l ongest piece of writing I've done in months, but I can work on fabric.

- The cats. They curl up on the bed with me when I'm napping, sleep with me when I'm watching a movie on Netflix (what a wonderful thing that is!) and generally keep me company. I find their warm, purring bodies comforting.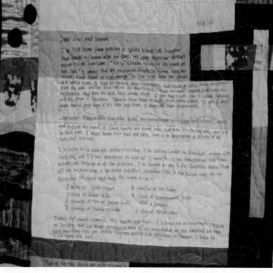

- Enough money. This would be so much harder if I was worrying about paying bills.

- My parents aren't alive. This would be so much harder if my parents were involved. I used to tell Alan, "If I'm really sick, don't tell my parents. Call them after I'm dead."

Isn't that awful? But it's the truth. My brother, on the other hand, has been very supportive. We talk about once a week, and this illness has deepened and confirmed the love and the bond that we share.

So there's very little cause for self-pity, and many, many reasons for gratitude. I think about a 30 year old single mother with breast cancer. How does she manage with kids, no husband, and the need to work in order to get her medical benefits? I have it easy compared to many women diagnosed with breast cancer.

One of the things I've loved about this experience is the way people have prayed for me. I'm on the list in Presbyterian churches and the local Jewish synagogue. My Hindu friends offer prayers for me at their temple in SLC. My boss, the associate provost, came over and gave me a Mormon blessing, oil on the head and all. I don't mind where the thoughts and prayers come from; they all work.

There'll be lessons to learn out of all this, but I don't know what they are yet. They're not likely to be as life changing as the Hodgkin's, but I expect there will be some sort of refining and honing.

I'm mostly at home these days, but we did make the decision to try to go away for a few days before each round of chemo. Just before I started the first chemo, we went down to Moab for a few days and stayed in a lovely cabin, tucked away in a quiet canyon. It was lovely to get away and hike (gently) in that slick rock country. Last week-end, we went south to St George for a few days before this second chemo.

On to other things: I'm not reading much, but I'm watching a lot of movies. I'll recommend just one to you: "The Triplets of Bellevue." It's a French cartoon about a devoted grandmother and a professional cyclist. The best character in it is the dog. It's a funny, clever and touching movie. Really wonderful.

I'm also addicted to the Showtime series, "Dexter." Erica suggested it to me, and I respect her taste in films and books, so I sent for it through Netflix. The premise sounds awful: it's about a serial killer who kills other serial killers. However, he has a code he works by: he only kills people who kill others. I know, it sounds bizarre, but it's cleverly written and acted, and the story line takes him to the edge all the time. It's ironic and funny.

And on Sunday, I turn 60. I'm so surprised to be that old and also delighted that I've made it this far. I well remember and cherish the celebration of my 50th birthday in Tucson, and I've never forgotten that amazing chocolate cake you made, Susan. I hope we'll be able to celebrate my 60th when I'm healthy.

I will hold a small potluck party for 5 women friends on April 21st, and Alan will organize something with his family for the 22nd. It will be low key, but I certainly want to celebrate reaching 60.

I'm reaching that stage in life when death is no longer an "if" but a "when," something I understood in my twenties when I had Hodgkins, but death is still a hard idea to get my mind round.

And now I'll comment on Susan's entry, focused so much on the idea of death. I suppose we're not sure about a "good" death. Tony used to quote Euripides, "Count no man happy till he dies," but I think that's BS. We have so little control over when or how we die, whereas we can make all sorts of choices about how we live. And what is a "good" death? Does that mean it's quick, like my uncle who dropped dead of a heart attack while walking the family dog? Or does it mean it's a long enough process to put everything in order and say goodbyes? I think of my mother's last couple of years which were bloody awful. I'd take the quick death any time. Or does it mean dying after living a long life? But what if you pack a lot into a short life, like the Bronte sisters, doesn't that count for more than a long but unmemorable life? I'm just not sure it's possible to know what a "good" death is.

Even with my history, I haven't dwelled much on death over the years. However, as I grow older, I think a lot about the aging process because, again, I have some choices to make. As I grow older, I want to honor my body even more than I already do with exercise and nutrition and kindness. I want to become more open-minded to difference. I want to be able to adapt cheerfully to change because it's coming whether I like it or not. I want to be more good humored, kinder to other people, more willing to let them be who they are. There's an art and a discipline to aging that I'm working to develop.

Love,

Judy

Chapter 5: Healing Quilts
Healing Quote Quilt

36" wide by 43" long

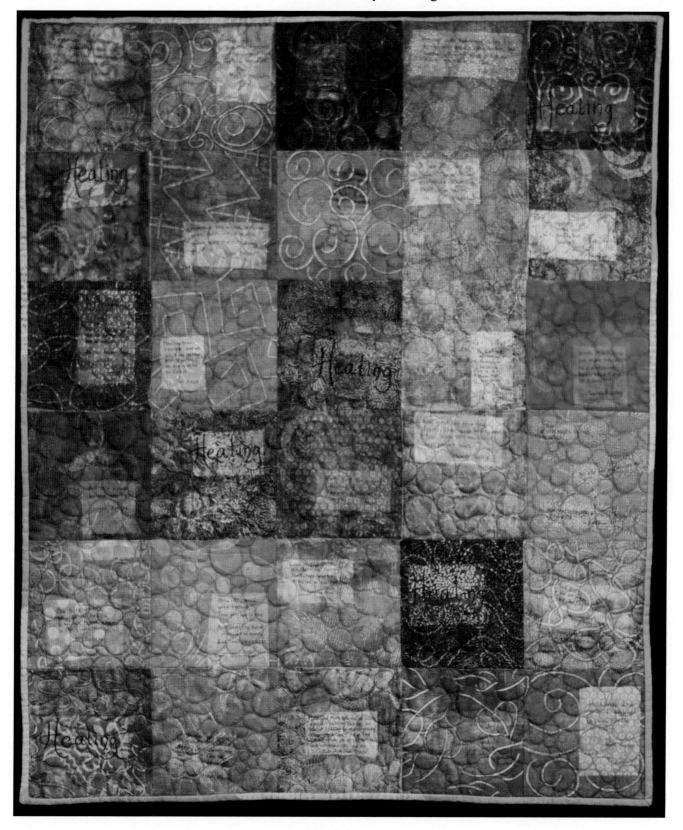

Chapter 5:   Healing Quilts

It took a long time to believe in my own healing. This first quilt in this section, "Healing Quotes," shows I still had little confidence in my recovery: I used other people's words rather than my own. However, it was an important first step.

My friend, Sue Stauffacher, sent me a series of collaged boards, each one containing a quote about healing. I used many of her quotes for the first quilt.

In the second quilt, "I'll Know I'm Healed When . . ." I finally used my own words to say what healing meant for me. This quilt explores what the new healthy me would look like. Some markers signal a return to what I could do before, such as working and exercise, and others reach to a new life after breast cancer. You'll notice I don't use the word, "cure." None of us are cured from the business of life, but we can craft healthy lives.

I made the fabric of both these quilts with gel plates and mono printing.

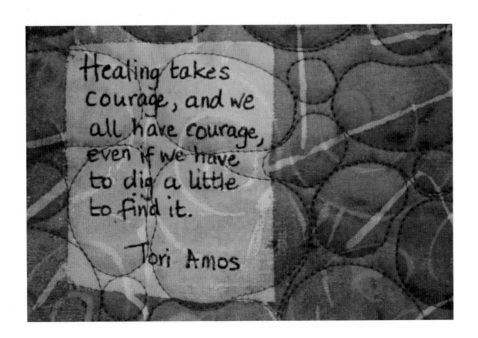

"Healing may not be so much about getting better as about letting go of everything that isn't you —all of the expectations, all of the beliefs — and becoming who you are. "   Rachel Naomi Remen

"There is more wisdom in your body than in your deepest philosophies.."
Friedrich Nietzsche

"Hold on to what is good even if it is a handful of earth." Hopi proverb

"Joy and sorrow are inseparable . . . Together they come, and when one sits alone with you, remember the other is asleep upon your bed."
Kahlil Gibran

"The body is not the measure of healing; peace is the measure. " Phyllis McGinley

"No one saves us but ourselves. No can and no one may. We ourselves must walk the path." The Buddha

"Although the world is filled with suffering, it is also filled with the overcoming of it. "
Helen Keller

"A jug fills drop by drop. The mind is everything. What you think, you become."

The Buddha

"Art is a wound turned into light." Georges Braque

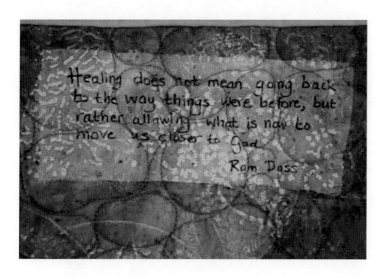

Healing does not mean going back to the way things were before, but rather allowing what is now to move us closer to God.
Ram Dass

"At the deepest level, the creative process and the healing process arise from a single source. When you are an artist, you are a healer."   Rachel Naomi Remen

"Nothing can bring you peace but yourself. " Emerson

"Believe nothing, no matter where you read it or who said it unless it agrees with your own reason or your own common sense."
The Buddha

"You can be an agent for healing another by simply by being present with them consciously and patiently." Sarah Fielding

I'll Know I'm Healed When . . .

26" wide by 39" long

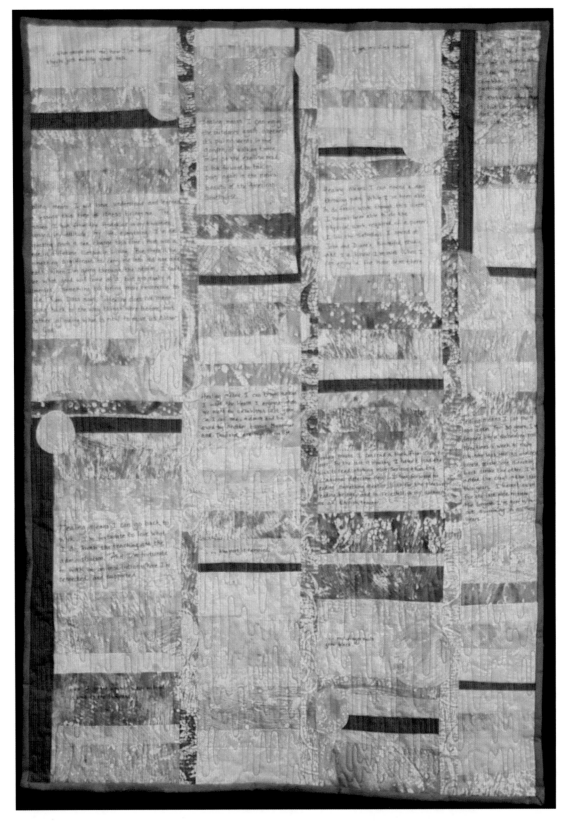

"I'll Know I'm Healed When . . ." was one of the last quilts I made to articulate all the ways I'd know when I was healthy. Here are some of my markers, inscribed on the quilt:

I'll know I'm healed when:

- . . People ask me how I'm doing, they'll just be making small talk.

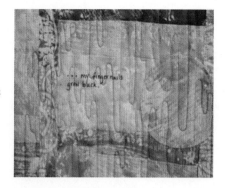

- . . . I can enjoy the outdoors again. Whether it's pulling weeds in the garden or walking three miles on the exercise trail, I look forward to taking part again in the natural beauty of the American Southwest.

- . . . I can spend a day throwing pots. While I've been able to do fabric work through this illness, I haven't been able to do the physical work required of a potter. I love the Saturdays I spend in John and Diane's Bountiful studio, and I'll know I'm well when I can enjoy a five hour stint there.

- . . . I can read a book from cover to cover. For the last nine months, I haven't had the focus to read anything more serious than the occasional detective novel. I look forward to reading something meatier, both for the pleasure reading brings, and to reestablish my authority as an English teacher.

- . . . I go for a whole week without a visit to the hospital.

- . . . I can go back to work. I'm fortunate to love what I do, both the teaching and the administration. And I'm fortunate to work at an institution where I'm respected and supported.

- . . . The port is removed.

- . . . My fingernails grow back.

- . . . I can travel again. I want the health I enjoyed when we went to Uzbekistan last year so I can see, admire and be awed by another culture. Myanmar and Thailand are high on my list.

- . . . I have understood and learned the lessons this time of illness brings me. The lessons I took from the Hodgkin's in my twenties changed my attitudes, my life, everything. I'm not expecting such a sea change this time: that was a once in a lifetime Lesson in Living. But there'll be something significant to carry me into old age and death. When I'm going through the storm, I can't see what good will come of it, but gradually it emerges, something to bring more reverence to life. Ram Dass says, "Healing does not mean going back to the ways things were before, but rather allowing what is now to move us closer to God."

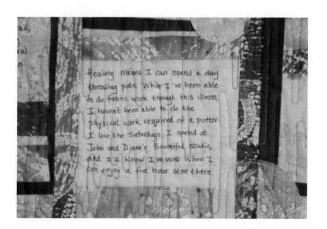

Chapter 6

The Chemo Quilt

I worked on this quilt, like many of the others in this book, as I sat in the chemo room for four or five hours every three weeks.

I wanted to visualize the chemo in my body. What did it do? How did it work? Fire was the metaphor that worked for me, both burning and purifying.

The colored beads show the cancer cells wandering around my body, and the white beads represent white blood cells. The smallest flame is filled only with white beads, in the hope that my body will eventually eliminate the cancer.

The background fabric for "Chemo" was dyed by my friend, Julie Nelson, who also wrote on the cloth. Her fabric represents my body at work, each part smoothly communicating with all the other parts.

This quilt won overall first prize in the biennial Lilly "Oncology on Canvas" competition, as well as first prize in the mixed media category, and first prize by someone with cancer category. (http://www.lillyoncologyoncanvas.com). $12,000 in prize money was donated in my name to the Utah chapter of Casting for Recovery. I attended their 2012 weekend retreat, offered to women who have had breast cancer, where we learned to fly fish as well as sharing our cancer stories, questions and answers with others who have been on this journey.

"Chemo" was published in the 2012 *Lilly Oncology on Canvas: Expressions of a Cancer Journey*, a book distributed to cancer centers across the country. The quilt now belongs to the Lilly Corporation.

Overall Winners

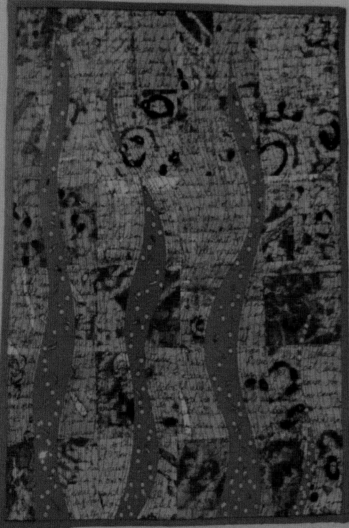

0074-1F 2032

CHEMO

*Mixed Media by a Person
Diagnosed with Cancer
Utah*

I was diagnosed with breast cancer in January 2012, and I'm currently halfway through chemotherapy. As a long time quilter, I've expressed my journey through my fabric work. I hand dye all my fabrics, starting with 100 percent white cotton.

This quilt shows the work of chemo as it flows through the port into my blood stream. The colored beads represent the chemo, and the white beads signify white blood cells helping my body move towards health. I visualize the future in the smallest plume on the right side of the quilt, a time when my blood stream will carry plenty of white blood cells—no chemo or cancer present.

I designed and made this quilt, using a combination of machine and hand stitching

Award Winner

**Best of Exhibition–
1st Prize Winner**

**Best Entry by a Person
Diagnosed with Cancer**

**Best Mixed Media by a Person
Diagnosed with Cancer**

Chapter 7:   Prompts and Questions for the Reader

Each quilt in this book invites the reader to consider her own experience:

What the Body Knew:

Were there signs before your diagnosis that you can now recognize?

Journal quilts:

How can you document your experience with cancer in a way that is meaningful to you?

What I Love About Life:

What do you love about your life?

It Takes a Village to Cure a Sick Person:

Who makes up your village of support?

Anna Quindlen Quote:

What's the difference between your experience day to day, and the way other people view you?

Daily Prayer:

What daily mantra, prayer or thought is helpful to you?

Words of Encouragement:

What words have been most encouraging to you?

Letter to Sue and Susan:

Who or what do you want to thank through your breast cancer experience?

Chemo:

How do you visualize your chemo or radiation treatment?

Healing Quote Quilt:

Can you find quotes about health and healing that seem particularly wise to you?

I'll Know I'm Healed When . . .

What does healing look like for you?

Chapter 8:   Textile Techniques

All the quilts are made from 100% PDF (prepared for dyeing) white cotton cloth, using the following techniques:

Dyeing and overdyeing: using Procion MX dyes. I start with the primary colors, red, yellow, and blue, and mix all my other colors from there.

Shibori : a Japanese technique for manipulating cloth before it's dyed in order to create patterns. We see the American version of this technique in tie-dyeing.

Improvisational screen printing: Using thickened dyes, I create a design on a screen that will last for four or five pulls. As the dye imprints on the fabric, the screen print changes.

Thermofax: a permanent screen burned into specially treated surface. A thermofax produces a sharp and detailed image unlike improvisational printing.

Discharging: Removing color out of dyed fabric with a thickened bleach product.

Stamping: I make my own stamps from small blocks of wood and sticky back foam.

Applique: I apply one fabric on top of another using a double fused product like Under Wonder.

Gel Plate mono printing: This is a jelly-like rectangle that holds an impression long enough to monoprint thickened dye or fabric paint.

I also use permanent fabric pens and beading on some quilts.

Chapter 9:   Exhibitions

The quilts in this book have been exhibited in a number of different places, including:

Home Machine Quilting Show, featured speaker, Salt Lake City, UT	May 2013
"40 Days and 40 Nights" solo show of the journal quilts in the	
Shaw Gallery at Weber State University.	October 2013
Machine Quilters Showcase, banquet speaker, Wichita, Kansas	April 2014
Art Access, Salt Lake City	January 2015
Machine Quilters Showcase, banquet speaker, Kansas City, Kansas	April 2014
Weber State University Student Gallery, Ogden, UT	February 2016

"Show and Tell" presentations on the breast cancer quilts:

Casting for Recovery, annual Utah retreat: opening night speaker.	2013,2014,2015
Weber County Senior Health Professionals, Roy, Utah	2013
Utah Quilt Study Group, Salt Lake City	2013

If you are interested in an exhibition and/or talk on these breast cancer quilts, please contact me at: jelsley@weber.edu

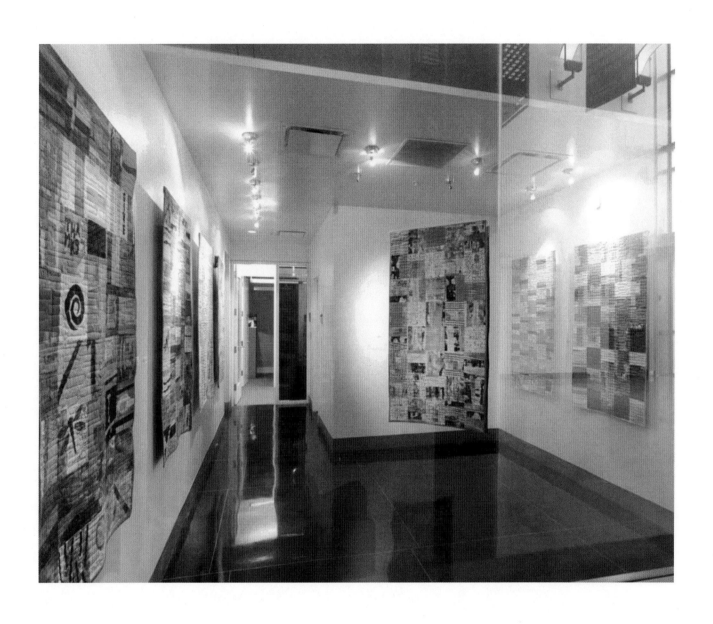

"40 Days and 40 Nights" solo show of the journal quilts
in the Shaw Gallery at Weber State University,
Ogden, Utah.   October 2013

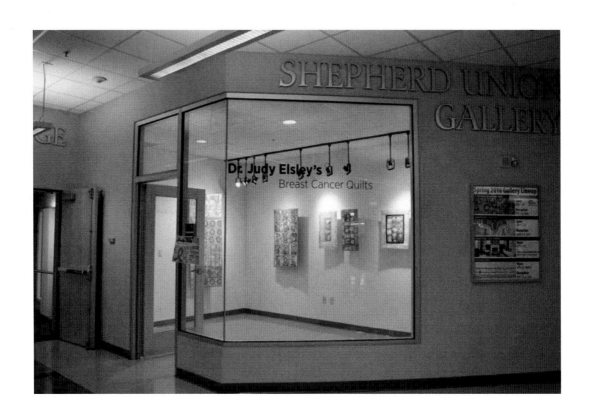

"Breast Cancer Quilts," solo show
in the Shepherd Union Gallery,
Weber State University Ogden, UT   February 2016

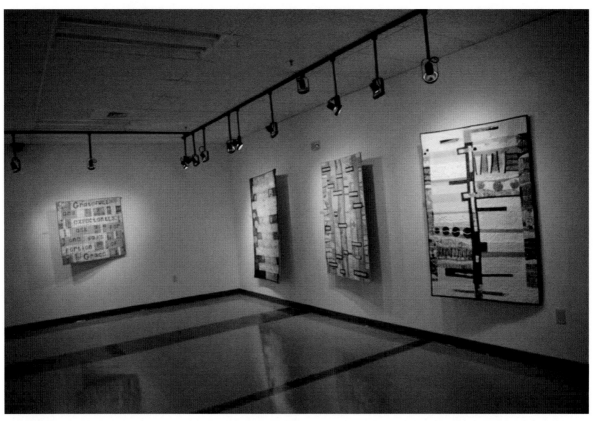

My Publications Related to Quilts and Quilting

Books:

Quilts As Text(ile)s: The Semiotics of Quilting. (A revision of my Ph.D. dissertation) Peter Lang Publications. 1996.

Quilt Culture: Tracing the Patterns. (An anthology of essays theorizing quilting) Edited with Cheryl Torsney, Professor at West Virginia University. University of Missouri Press, 1994.

Articles:

"Chemo," Lilly Oncology on Canvas: Expressions of a Cancer Journey. Best of Exhibition, 1st Prize Winner; Best Entry by a Person Diagnosed with Cancer; Best Mixed Media by a Person Diagnosed with Cancer. 2012.

"Trusting the Process: The Creative Links Between Writing and Quilting," Textile Perspectives, British Quilting Guild. Issue 49, Summer 2010. Ps. 14-16.

"Pens and Needles: Writing About Quilts." Textile Perspectives, British Quilting Guild. Issue 47, Summer 2009. June 2009.

"Annotated Bibliography of a Selection of Children's Books Featuring Quilts and Quilters." Blanket Statements, issue 71, Winter 2003. P. 13.

"Tell Me a Story: Cultural Values in Quilt Literature." Uncoverings: Journal of the American Quilt Study Group, Vol. 23. Lincoln, Nebraska: American Quilt Study Group, 2002. 65-80.

"Nothing can be sole or whole that has not been rent": Fragmentation in the Quilt and The Color Purple. Reprinted in Critical Essays on Alice Walker, edited by Ikenna Dieke. Westport, Connecticut: Greenwood Press, 1999. 163-170

"A Stitch in Crime: Quilt Detective Novels." Uncoverings: Journal of the American Quilt Study Group, Vol. 19, 1998. 137-153.

"An AIDS Patchwork: personal essay." Weber Studies. Vol. 13, No. 3, Fall 1996. 65-74.

"Making Critical Connections in Quilt Scholarship." Uncoverings: Journal of the American Quilt Study Group, Vol. 16, 1995. 229-243.

"The Color Purple and the Poetics of Fragmentation," in Quilt Culture: Tracing the   Pattern. Ed. Cheryl Torsney and Judy Elsley. University of Missouri Press, 1994. 68-83.

"The Smithsonian Controversy: Cultural Dislocation." Uncoverings: Journal of the American Quilt Study Group, vol.14, 1993. 119-136.

"Bound By Tradition," essay for Bound By Tradition Quilt Exhibition Catalog, sponsored by the Utah Humanities Council. December 1993.

""For Want of a Purse: Eliza Calvert Hall's Short Story "Aunt Jane of Kentucky." Legacy: A Journal of American Women Writers. Vol.9, No. 2, 1992. 119-127.

"Nothing Can Be Sole or Whole That Has Not Been Rent: Fragmentation in the Quilt and The Color Purple." Weber Studies: An Interdisciplinary Humanities Journal. Spring/Summer 1992, Vol. 9 No. 2. 71-81.

"Laughter as Feminine Power in The Color Purple and A Question of Silence." New Perspectives on Women and Comedy. Ed. Regina Barreca. Gordon and Breach: Gender and Culture Series, Vol. 5, 1992. 193-200.

"The Rhetoric of the NAMES Project AIDS Quilt: Reading the Text(ile)." AIDS: The Literary Response. Ed. Emmanuel Nelson. Twayne, 1992. 187-196.

"Uncovering Eliza Calvert Hall." Encyclia: The Journal of Utah Academy of Sciences, Arts and Letters. Vol 68, 1991. 155-172.

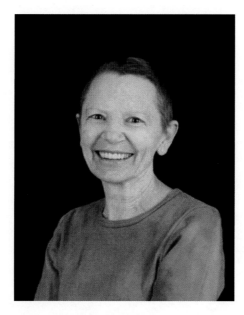

Growing my hair back after chemo

I was born and raised in England. After moving to the U.S. in 1979, I completed an M.A. at the University of Nevada in Las Vegas in 1985, and a Ph.D. in English Literature at the University of Arizona in Tucson in 1990.

Quilting has been the subject of many of my published articles. I have written about quilt related literature; quilts in contemporary culture; and the place of academics in quilt scholarship. I have also co-edited a book of academic essays on quilting: *Quilt Culture: Tracing the Patterns,* published by the University of Missouri Press in 1994. A rewritten version of my dissertation was published by Peter Lang Press under the title, *Quilts as Text(ile)s.*

I also write and publish personal essays. In 1997, Jumping Cholla Press published my book of personal essays, *Getting Comfortable,* about living in the American West. The book is now available through Amazon.

I taught in the English Department at Weber State University from 1990 to 2016 when I retired. During my tenure, I also directed a number of programs, most recently the university's Honors Program.

Made in the USA
Columbia, SC
29 November 2019

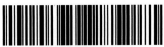

84018572R00049